Disease Detectives: Unraveling the Secrets of Plant Pathology for Students

Astrid Jensen

Copyright © [2023]

Title: Disease Detectives: Unraveling the Secrets of Plant Pathology for Students

Author's: Astrid Jensen.

This book was printed and published by [Publisher's: Astrid Jensen] in [2023]

ISBN:

TABLE OF CONTENTS

Chapter 3: Identifying Plant Diseases   35

Chapter 4: Causes and Transmission of Plant Diseases 69

Chapter 5: Prevention and Control of Plant Diseases 109

Chapter 6: Disease Detection and Surveillance 160

Chapter 7: Case Studies in Plant Pathology 178

Chapter 8: Future Directions in Plant Pathology   205

Chapter 9: Conclusion and Key Takeaways   217

Chapter 1: Introduction to Plant Pathology

The Importance of Plant Health

Plants are an essential part of our planet's ecosystem, providing us with food, oxygen, and numerous other resources. However, just like humans and animals, plants are also susceptible to diseases. Understanding the importance of plant health and the field of plant pathology is crucial for students interested in the field of botany.

Plant health refers to the overall well-being of plants, including their ability to resist diseases, pests, and environmental stresses. Healthy plants not only yield higher crop production but also contribute to a balanced and sustainable environment. As students delve into the world of botany, they will realize that maintaining plant health is of utmost importance for the future of agriculture and the planet.

Plant pathology is the study of plant diseases and the science behind their prevention, diagnosis, and treatment. Disease detectives, or plant pathologists, play a crucial role in identifying and managing plant diseases to ensure the health and productivity of crops. By understanding the causes, symptoms, and transmission of plant diseases, students can help protect plants from harmful pathogens and work towards sustainable agriculture.

Plant diseases can have devastating effects, leading to significant yield losses, economic hardships, and even famine in some regions. By learning about plant health, students gain the knowledge and skills necessary to prevent and manage these diseases effectively. They can recognize early signs of disease, implement proper disease management techniques, and develop innovative strategies to combat plant pathogens in a sustainable manner.

Moreover, plant health is not only essential for agriculture but also impacts the natural environment. Healthy plants contribute to the biodiversity of ecosystems, supporting a wide range of organisms, including insects, birds, and mammals. By preserving plant health, students can contribute to the conservation of natural habitats and promote sustainable practices.

In conclusion, the importance of plant health cannot be overstated. As students interested in botany, understanding plant diseases and their management is crucial for a sustainable future. By becoming disease detectives, students can contribute to the preservation of plant health, ensuring food security, environmental balance, and the well-being of our planet.

What is Plant Pathology?

Plant pathology is a fascinating field of study that explores the causes, development, and prevention of diseases in plants. It is a branch of botany that focuses on understanding and managing plant diseases, which can have devastating effects on agricultural crops, forests, and natural ecosystems.

In simple terms, plant pathology investigates the interactions between plants and the pathogens that infect them. These pathogens can include fungi, bacteria, viruses, nematodes, and other microorganisms. By studying these interactions, plant pathologists aim to find ways to control and prevent the spread of diseases, ensuring the health and productivity of plants.

One of the primary goals of plant pathology is to identify and diagnose plant diseases accurately. This involves observing and analyzing symptoms, such as wilting, discoloration, or abnormal growth patterns, to determine the cause of the illness. Plant pathologists use various techniques, such as microscopy, molecular biology, and laboratory testing, to identify the specific pathogens responsible for the disease.

Understanding the biology and life cycles of plant pathogens is another crucial aspect of plant pathology. By studying how pathogens infect and reproduce within plants, scientists can develop strategies to interrupt their life cycles and prevent further spread. This knowledge helps in the development of effective control measures, including the use of resistant plant varieties, cultural practices, biological controls, and chemical treatments.

Plant pathology also plays a vital role in protecting the environment and ensuring food security. By studying plant diseases, scientists can assess the risks associated with new and emerging pathogens, as well as the impact of climate change on disease prevalence. This information enables them to develop sustainable strategies for disease management, reducing the reliance on chemical pesticides and promoting environmentally friendly practices.

As students of botany, learning about plant pathology opens up a world of opportunities. It allows you to explore the intricate relationships between plants and pathogens, discover innovative solutions to combat diseases, and contribute to the preservation and improvement of our natural resources. Whether you aspire to become a plant pathologist, a plant breeder, or an environmental scientist, understanding the principles of plant pathology is essential for a successful career in the field of botany.

The Role of Disease Detectives

In the field of botany, disease detectives play a crucial role in unraveling the secrets of plant pathology. These dedicated individuals are scientists who investigate and study plant diseases, working tirelessly to understand the causes, effects, and methods of prevention or control. Disease detectives are the unsung heroes of the plant world, fighting against destructive pathogens that threaten crops, forests, and the overall health of our environment.

One of the primary responsibilities of disease detectives is to identify and diagnose plant diseases. They possess an in-depth knowledge of plant anatomy and physiology, allowing them to recognize the symptoms and signs of various diseases. By observing changes in leaf color, growth patterns, or the presence of fungi or bacteria, disease detectives can pinpoint the specific pathogen responsible for the plant's decline. This diagnostic expertise is vital in developing effective control strategies and preventing the spread of diseases.

Once a disease is identified, disease detectives work to understand its causes and develop methods for prevention or control. They conduct experiments and research to determine the mode of transmission, environmental factors that favor disease development, and potential treatments. Disease detectives collaborate with other scientists, including geneticists, agronomists, and ecologists, to explore innovative solutions and develop resistant plant varieties. Their work often involves field surveys, laboratory experiments, and the use of advanced technologies like DNA sequencing to unravel the mysteries of plant pathology.

In addition to research and diagnosis, disease detectives also play a crucial role in educating and raising awareness among students and the general public. Through workshops, seminars, and publications, they share their knowledge and findings, helping others understand the importance of plant health and the impact of diseases on food security and the environment. By promoting good agricultural practices, disease detectives empower farmers and gardeners to prevent and manage diseases effectively.

As students interested in botany, you have the opportunity to become disease detectives yourselves. Pursuing a career in plant pathology can open doors to exciting research, discovery, and the chance to make a real difference in the world. By becoming disease detectives, you can contribute to the development of sustainable agriculture, protect natural ecosystems, and ensure that future generations have access to healthy and abundant plant resources.

So, if you are passionate about plants, curious about the unseen world of pathogens, and eager to unravel the secrets of plant diseases, consider a career as a disease detective. The world needs your expertise, dedication, and passion to ensure the health and prosperity of our precious botanical treasures.

Chapter 2: Understanding Plant Diseases

What are Plant Diseases?

Plants, just like humans and animals, can fall prey to diseases. These diseases, known as plant diseases, are caused by various agents such as fungi, bacteria, viruses, and other microorganisms. They can affect different parts of a plant, including leaves, stems, roots, flowers, and fruits, leading to stunted growth, reduced yield, or even death. Understanding plant diseases is crucial for students studying botany as it helps them comprehend the complex world of plants and the challenges they face.

Plant diseases can manifest in several ways, each with its own set of symptoms. Some common symptoms include wilting, yellowing of leaves, spots or lesions on the foliage, rotting of roots or fruits, and abnormal growth patterns. These symptoms can vary depending on the specific pathogen causing the disease and the affected plant species. By learning to recognize these symptoms, students can identify potential diseases and take appropriate measures to manage or prevent them.

Fungi are one of the most common causes of plant diseases. They reproduce through spores and thrive in damp and warm environments. For example, powdery mildew is a fungal disease characterized by a white powdery coating on the leaves, while rust fungi create reddish-brown pustules on the plant surface. Bacterial diseases, on the other hand, are caused by specific bacteria that invade the plant tissues, causing lesions and tissue decay.

Viruses are another significant group of plant pathogens. They are tiny infectious agents that cannot replicate on their own and rely on host cells for reproduction. Viral diseases can be challenging to manage, as they can spread rapidly through insect vectors or contaminated tools. Some viral diseases result in mottled or distorted leaves, stunted growth, or abnormal fruit development.

Students studying botany must also understand the importance of plant disease management. This involves implementing preventive measures such as selecting disease-resistant plant varieties, practicing proper sanitation, and ensuring optimal plant nutrition and care. In some cases, chemical treatments may be necessary to control or suppress diseases, but sustainable and environmentally friendly approaches should always be prioritized.

By delving into the world of plant diseases, students gain insight into the delicate balance between plants and their pathogens. They learn about the complex interactions between plants and microorganisms and how these interactions shape ecosystems. Ultimately, this knowledge equips them to become disease detectives, unraveling the secrets of plant pathology and contributing to the field of botany in their future careers.

Common Types of Plant Diseases

In the exciting world of botany, understanding plant diseases is paramount to the health and vitality of plants. As budding botanists, it is essential to unravel the secrets of plant pathology and learn about the common types of plant diseases that can affect our green friends. This subchapter will introduce you, students of botany, to some of the most prevalent plant diseases.

1. Fungal Diseases: Fungi are the most common culprits when it comes to plant diseases. They can cause leaf spots, root rots, and wilts. Some well-known fungal diseases include powdery mildew, which forms a white powdery coating on plant leaves, and rust, which appears as orange or brown spots on leaves and stems.

2. Bacterial Diseases: Bacteria can wreak havoc on plants by causing diseases such as bacterial blight and crown gall. Bacterial blight leads to brown spots on leaves and can cause defoliation. Crown gall causes abnormal growths, or galls, on plant stems and roots.

3. Viral Diseases: Viruses are tiny infectious agents that can cause a range of diseases in plants. Symptoms can vary widely, from mosaic patterns on leaves to stunted growth. Some common viral diseases include tomato mosaic virus and cucumber mosaic virus.

4. Nematode Diseases: Nematodes are microscopic roundworms that can damage plant roots, affecting their growth and nutrient uptake. Symptoms of nematode infestation include stunted growth, wilting, and yellowing leaves.

5. Parasitic Plant Diseases: Parasitic plants, such as dodder and mistletoe, can attach themselves to host plants and sap their nutrients. These parasites weaken the host plant and can even cause its death if left untreated.

Understanding these common types of plant diseases is crucial for proper plant care and maintenance. By recognizing the symptoms and identifying the causal agents, you can take appropriate measures to prevent or treat these diseases. Prevention strategies may include maintaining proper sanitation, using disease-resistant plant varieties, and practicing crop rotation.

In the field of botany, being a disease detective is essential. By unraveling the secrets of plant pathology, we can protect and nurture our beloved plants. So, students of botany, let us delve deeper into the fascinating world of plant diseases and uncover the solutions to keep our green friends healthy and thriving.

Fungal Diseases

Fungal diseases are a significant concern in the field of botany. They can affect plants of all kinds, from towering trees in the rainforest to delicate flowers in your backyard garden. Understanding these diseases is crucial for students interested in botany, as they play a vital role in plant pathology.

Fungi are a diverse group of organisms that can cause a wide range of diseases in plants. They are microscopic in size and can be found almost everywhere in the environment. While most fungi are harmless to plants, some can become pathogens and cause serious damage. These pathogens invade plant tissues, disrupting their normal functioning and leading to diseases.

There are several types of fungal diseases that students should be aware of. One common type is called powdery mildew, which appears as a white powdery substance on the leaves, stems, and flowers of infected plants. This disease can weaken the plant, making it more susceptible to other infections. Another well-known fungal disease is rust, characterized by orange or brown spots that develop on leaves and other plant parts. Rust can cause defoliation and reduce the plant's ability to photosynthesize.

Students studying botany must also be familiar with the devastating effects of fungal diseases on crops. One example is the infamous Irish potato famine, which was caused by a fungal disease called late blight. This disease destroyed potato crops across Ireland, leading to widespread famine and the loss of millions of lives. Understanding the mechanisms behind such outbreaks can help students develop strategies to prevent and manage similar diseases in the future.

Preventing and managing fungal diseases is a critical aspect of plant pathology. Students should learn about the different methods used to control these diseases, such as cultural practices, genetic resistance, and the use of fungicides. By implementing these strategies, farmers and gardeners can minimize the impact of fungal diseases on their crops and plants.

In conclusion, fungal diseases are a significant concern in the field of botany. Students interested in plant pathology must familiarize themselves with the different types of fungal diseases, their effects on plants, and the strategies used to prevent and manage them. By understanding these aspects, students can contribute to the development of sustainable practices in agriculture and horticulture, ensuring the health and productivity of plants for future generations.

Introduction:
In the fascinating world of botany, plants are not immune to various diseases. Just like humans and animals, plants can also fall victim to infections caused by fungi. These fungal diseases can have profound effects on the health and vitality of plants, often leading to stunted growth, reduced productivity, and even death. In this subchapter, we will dive into the world of fungal diseases, exploring their causes, symptoms, and potential management strategies.

Understanding Fungal Diseases:
Fungal diseases in plants are caused by various types of fungi, including molds, mildews, and yeasts. These microscopic organisms

often thrive in warm and humid environments, making plants susceptible to infections in such conditions. Fungi can infect any part of a plant, including leaves, stems, fruits, and roots.

Common   Fungal   Diseases:
1. Powdery Mildew: This disease manifests as a powdery white coating on the leaves and stems of plants, inhibiting their ability to carry out photosynthesis. Powdery mildew can affect a wide range of plant species and is typically prevalent in cool and dry climates.

2. Rust: Rust diseases cause reddish-brown or orange-colored pustules to appear on leaves, stems, and fruits. These pustules contain fungal spores that can spread rapidly, leading to defoliation and reduced plant vigor. Rust diseases are commonly found in moist environments.

3. Fusarium Wilt: This devastating disease affects the vascular system of plants, obstructing the flow of water and nutrients. Plants infected with Fusarium wilt often display wilting, yellowing, and stunted growth. This disease can be challenging to manage once established.

Management   and   Prevention:
Preventing and managing fungal diseases in plants requires a multi-faceted approach. Here are some strategies that can help:

1. Cultural Practices: Maintaining good plant hygiene, such as removing and destroying infected plant parts, can prevent the spread of fungal diseases. Proper watering techniques and adequate spacing between plants can also reduce humidity levels and minimize the risk of infection.

2. Fungicides: In severe cases, fungicides can be used to control fungal diseases. However, it is essential to choose and apply these chemicals responsibly, following the instructions provided.

3. Resistant Varieties: Plant breeders have developed cultivars that are resistant to specific fungal diseases. Choosing these resistant varieties can significantly reduce the risk of infection.

Conclusion:

Fungal diseases pose a significant threat to the health and productivity of plants. By understanding the causes, symptoms, and management strategies of these diseases, students with an interest in botany can contribute to the prevention and control of these infections. By implementing proper cultural practices, utilizing effective fungicides when necessary, and selecting resistant plant varieties, we can help protect our precious plants from the devastating impact of fungal diseases.

Bacterial Diseases

Bacteria are microscopic organisms that can cause a wide range of diseases in plants. These diseases, known as bacterial diseases, can have a significant impact on plant health and productivity. In this subchapter, we will explore some common bacterial diseases that affect plants and learn about the strategies employed by disease detectives in unraveling their secrets.

One of the most well-known bacterial diseases is fire blight, which affects a variety of fruit trees such as apple, pear, and quince. Fire blight is caused by the bacterium Erwinia amylovora and can cause severe damage to orchards. Infected plants display symptoms such as wilting, blackening of stems, and a scorched appearance, hence the name "fire blight." Disease detectives study the pathogen's life cycle, transmission methods, and environmental factors to develop effective control strategies.

Another significant bacterial disease is bacterial leaf spot, which affects a wide range of plants including tomatoes, peppers, and lettuce. This disease is caused by various bacteria, such as Xanthomonas spp. and Pseudomonas spp. Infected plants show characteristic leaf spots that start as small, water-soaked lesions and later develop into dark, necrotic areas. Disease detectives investigate factors such as host susceptibility, environmental conditions, and cultural practices to develop management strategies.

In addition to these specific diseases, there are numerous other bacterial pathogens that affect different parts of plants, including the roots, stems, and leaves. These pathogens can cause symptoms like wilting, cankers, and gumming. Disease detectives use various tools and techniques to identify and characterize these pathogens, including microscopy, DNA analysis, and laboratory experiments.

Understanding bacterial diseases is crucial for students studying botany as it helps them develop insights into the complex interactions between plants and pathogens. By learning about the symptoms, causes, and management strategies of bacterial diseases, students can contribute to the field of plant pathology and help protect our agricultural systems.

In conclusion, bacterial diseases pose a significant threat to plant health and can have severe economic consequences. Disease detectives play a crucial role in unraveling the secrets of bacterial diseases, studying their causes, transmission methods, and management strategies. By delving into the world of plant pathology, students interested in botany can contribute to the understanding and control of bacterial diseases, ultimately helping to safeguard our plant resources.

Bacteria are microscopic organisms that can cause a variety of diseases in plants. As students of botany, it is essential to understand the impact of bacterial diseases on plants and their role in plant pathology. In this subchapter, we will unravel the secrets behind bacterial diseases and their effects on plants.

Bacteria are single-celled organisms that can be found everywhere in our environment, including the soil, water, and even on the surface of plants. While many bacteria are harmless, some can be pathogenic, meaning they can cause diseases in plants. These pathogenic bacteria invade the plant's tissues, disrupting their normal functioning and causing visible symptoms.

One common bacterial disease is bacterial spot, which affects a wide range of plants, including tomatoes, peppers, and citrus trees. This disease manifests as dark, water-soaked lesions on leaves, stems, and fruits. Bacterial spot can reduce crop yield and quality, making it a significant concern for farmers and gardeners. Another well-known bacterial disease is fire blight, which primarily affects trees in the Rosaceae family, such as apple and pear trees. Fire blight causes wilting, blackening, and a scorched appearance of blossoms, branches, and fruit.

Understanding the spread and management of bacterial diseases is crucial for botany students. Bacteria can be transmitted through various means, including contaminated soil, water, tools, and even insects. By practicing good sanitation and hygiene, such as cleaning tools and avoiding overwatering, plant pathologists can help prevent the spread of bacterial diseases. Additionally, the use of disease-resistant plant varieties and implementing cultural practices like crop rotation can greatly reduce the impact of bacterial diseases.

Research plays a vital role in understanding and combating bacterial diseases. Scientists are constantly studying the pathogens, their interaction with plants, and developing new strategies for disease control. By staying up-to-date with the latest research and advancements, botany students can contribute to the field of plant pathology and help find innovative solutions to combat bacterial diseases.

In conclusion, bacterial diseases pose a significant threat to plants and can cause severe damage to crops and natural ecosystems. As students of botany, it is essential to understand the nature of bacterial diseases, their effects on plants, and the strategies for disease management. By acquiring this knowledge, we can contribute to the field of plant pathology and play our part in unraveling the secrets of bacterial diseases.

Viral Diseases

Viruses are microscopic organisms that can cause various diseases in plants, just like they do in animals and humans. In this subchapter, we will explore the world of viral diseases that affect plants, and how scientists in the field of plant pathology work to unravel their secrets.

Viral diseases in plants can be devastating, leading to stunted growth, reduced yield, and even death of the infected plant. These diseases are caused by plant viruses, which are tiny particles made up of genetic material surrounded by a protein coat. They cannot reproduce or survive outside a living host, and they infect plants by invading their cells.

One of the most famous viral diseases is the Tobacco mosaic virus (TMV), which affects tobacco plants. TMV causes a mosaic pattern of light and dark green on the leaves, along with curling and distortion. This virus can also infect other plants like tomatoes, peppers, and cucumbers.

Another viral disease that affects plants is the Potato virus Y (PVY), which primarily affects potatoes. PVY causes various symptoms, including mosaic patterns on leaves, stunted growth, and reduced tuber quality. This disease can significantly impact potato production and result in economic losses.

Plant pathologists study viral diseases to understand how they spread, how they affect plants, and how to control and prevent their spread. They use various techniques, such as molecular biology, to identify and characterize viruses, and develop strategies to manage them.

For example, plant pathologists can employ techniques like tissue culturing and heat therapy to produce virus-free plants, which can then be used for propagation. They also study the vectors that transmit viruses, such as aphids or whiteflies, and develop methods to control these vectors.

Understanding viral diseases is crucial for the field of botany as it helps botanists develop disease-resistant plant varieties through breeding or genetic engineering. By studying viral diseases, students interested in botany can contribute to the development of sustainable agricultural practices and help protect plant health.

In conclusion, viral diseases pose significant threats to plants, affecting their growth and overall productivity. Through the efforts of plant pathologists, scientists are unraveling the secrets of viral diseases, which is crucial for developing effective control strategies. By learning about viral diseases, students interested in botany can play a vital role in protecting plants and ensuring a sustainable future for agriculture.

In the fascinating world of plant pathology, one of the most intriguing topics is viral diseases. Viruses, which are incredibly tiny particles that cannot be seen with the naked eye, can have a profound impact on plant health and the overall ecosystem. In this subchapter, we will explore the secrets of viral diseases and their significance in the field of botany.

Viruses are unique infectious agents that rely on living organisms, such as plants, to replicate and spread. Similar to how a cold virus can make you sick, plant viruses can cause diseases that affect growth, development, and productivity. These diseases can manifest in various ways, including stunted growth, leaf discoloration, or even complete plant death.

Understanding viral diseases is crucial for botanists and plant pathologists, as it allows them to develop strategies to prevent and manage outbreaks. By studying how viruses infect plants, scientists can identify potential vectors, such as insects or nematodes, which transmit the virus from one plant to another. This knowledge helps in implementing effective control measures, like using insecticides or resistant plant varieties.

Furthermore, viral diseases can have significant implications for agriculture and food security. Crop plants, such as wheat, rice, or tomatoes, are susceptible to viral infections, which can lead to substantial yield losses. By learning about different viral diseases, students interested in botany can contribute to developing resistant plant varieties or innovative control methods, ensuring a sustainable and secure food supply for future generations.

In this subchapter, we will delve into the various types of viral diseases that affect plants, including mosaic viruses, leaf curl viruses, and necrotic viruses. We will explore their symptoms, transmission methods, and the specific plants they target. Additionally, we will discuss the innovative techniques used by plant pathologists to detect and identify viruses, such as serological tests, nucleic acid-based diagnostic methods, and advanced microscopy techniques.

To truly unravel the secrets of viral diseases, we will also explore the fascinating world of viral genomics and how it has revolutionized our understanding of plant-virus interactions. By studying the genetic makeup of both viruses and plants, scientists can gain insights into how viruses evolve, adapt, and overcome plant defenses, paving the way for the development of new strategies to combat viral diseases.

Whether you are a budding botanist or simply curious about the intricate world of plant pathology, this subchapter will take you on an exciting journey through the realm of viral diseases. Get ready to uncover the hidden secrets and mysteries behind these microscopic yet powerful pathogens that shape the world of botany.

Nematode Diseases

Nematode diseases are a significant concern in the field of botany, as they cause widespread damage to plants and crops. Nematodes are microscopic, worm-like organisms that live in the soil and feed on plant roots. They can infect various parts of a plant, including the roots, stems, leaves, and even the seeds. These tiny pests are responsible for significant yield losses in agriculture and can have a detrimental impact on plant health.

Nematode diseases are challenging to detect because the symptoms they cause are often similar to those caused by other plant pathogens or environmental factors. However, there are several signs that can help identify the presence of nematodes, such as stunted growth, yellowing or wilting of leaves, root galls, and reduced yields. It is crucial for botany students to be familiar with these symptoms to effectively diagnose and manage nematode diseases.

Prevention and management of nematode diseases involve several strategies. Crop rotation is an essential practice that helps disrupt the nematode life cycle and reduce their populations in the soil. By planting different crops in successive seasons, the nematodes that rely on specific host plants are deprived of their food source, leading to a decline in their numbers. Additionally, resistant plant varieties are available for some nematode species, which can be an effective means of control.

Chemical control methods, such as nematicides, are also used to manage nematode diseases. However, these should be used judiciously and in accordance with recommended guidelines, as they can have adverse effects on the environment and beneficial organisms. Integrated pest management (IPM) practices, which combine multiple strategies, including biological control and cultural practices, are considered the most sustainable approach to nematode disease management.

Botany students must also understand the importance of maintaining healthy soil conditions to prevent nematode infestations. Proper soil fertility, pH levels, and organic matter content contribute to vigorous plant growth and can reduce the susceptibility of plants to nematode diseases.

In conclusion, nematode diseases pose a significant threat to plants and crops, causing substantial economic losses. Botany students need to be aware of the signs and symptoms of nematode infestations and be equipped with the knowledge of prevention and management strategies. By incorporating sustainable practices and adopting integrated pest management approaches, students can contribute to the effective control of nematode diseases and ensure the health and productivity of plants.

Nematodes are microscopic, worm-like organisms that can cause significant damage to plants. In this subchapter, we will explore the various nematode diseases that affect plants and how they impact the field of botany.

Nematodes are found in almost every habitat on Earth and can infect a wide range of plant species. They are particularly harmful to crops, causing devastating losses in agricultural production worldwide. These tiny pests invade plant roots, feeding on the plant's cells and extracting nutrients, leading to stunted growth, wilting, and even death.

One of the most notorious nematode diseases is root-knot nematode. These microscopic pests form galls or knots on the roots of infected plants, impairing their ability to absorb water and nutrients from the soil. This disease affects a wide range of plants, including vegetables, fruits, and ornamental plants. Students studying botany should be aware of the symptoms of root-knot nematode infestation and its impact on plant health.

Another common nematode disease is cyst nematode. Unlike root-knot nematodes, cyst nematodes do not form visible galls on plant roots. Instead, they create cysts, protective structures that house their eggs. These cysts can survive in the soil for many years, making it difficult to control this disease. Cyst nematodes are a significant threat to important crops such as potatoes, soybeans, and wheat, and understanding their life cycle and management strategies is crucial for botany students interested in crop science.

Nematodes can also transmit viral diseases to plants. Some nematodes act as vectors, carrying plant viruses from one host to another. This can have a devastating impact on agricultural production, as viruses can cause severe damage to crops, leading to yield losses. Botany students should learn about the role of nematodes in spreading plant viruses and the importance of implementing effective management strategies to prevent disease transmission.

In conclusion, nematode diseases pose a significant threat to plant health and agricultural productivity. Understanding the impact of nematodes on plants is crucial for botany students interested in plant pathology and crop science. By recognizing the symptoms of nematode diseases and implementing effective management strategies, students can contribute to the development of sustainable solutions to combat these microscopic pests and safeguard our food supply.

Chapter 3: Identifying Plant Diseases

Recognizing Symptoms of Plant Diseases

In the fascinating world of botany, the study of plant diseases holds a crucial place. As students of this captivating field, it is essential for us to recognize the symptoms of plant diseases. By being able to identify these symptoms, we can take timely action to prevent further damage and save our beloved plants.

Plant diseases can manifest in various ways, often showing visible signs on leaves, stems, flowers, and fruits. One common symptom is the appearance of spots or discoloration on the leaves. These spots can be of different colors, such as brown, yellow, black, or even white. Paying close attention to any unusual markings on leaves can be a key factor in detecting plant diseases.

Another symptom to watch out for is wilting or drooping of the plant. If a plant suddenly starts to lose its turgidity and the leaves become limp, it could be an indication of disease. It is important to differentiate between wilting due to lack of water or nutrients and wilting caused by infections or pathogens.

Abnormal growth patterns are also significant indicators of plant diseases. For instance, if a plant starts to exhibit stunted growth, where it remains smaller than expected or fails to reach its full potential, it could be suffering from a disease. Additionally, distorted or misshapen leaves, stems, or flowers can also be a sign of infection.

Cankers, which are localized dead areas on stems or branches, are another symptom to be aware of. These cankers often appear as sunken, discolored patches and can lead to severe damage if left untreated. Bark splitting or peeling may accompany cankers, further emphasizing the presence of a disease.

Lastly, the presence of pests or insects on plants can be an indirect symptom of disease. Some insects, like aphids or whiteflies, are attracted to diseased plants. By observing the presence of these pests, we can infer that a plant might be suffering from an underlying disease.

As botany students, developing the skill to recognize symptoms of plant diseases is vital for our understanding of plant pathology. By honing this ability, we not only become more capable of diagnosing plant diseases, but also play a crucial role in preventing the spread of infections and protecting the health of plants. Remember, early detection is the key to successful disease management, and by being vigilant observers, we can become efficient disease detectives in the realm of botany.

As budding botanists, it is crucial for students to learn how to identify and recognize the symptoms of plant diseases. By doing so, you can become skilled disease detectives and help unravel the secrets of plant pathology. In this chapter, we will explore the various signs and symptoms that indicate the presence of plant diseases, equipping you with the knowledge needed to keep your plants healthy and thriving.

One of the most common symptoms of plant diseases is discoloration. Keep an eye out for leaves that turn yellow, brown, or develop unusual spots. Such discoloration can be indicative of nutrient deficiencies, fungal or bacterial infections, or viral diseases. Additionally, wilting or drooping leaves are often a sign of diseased plants. Wilting can occur due to excessive watering, lack of water, or even insect infestations.

Another symptom to watch out for is the presence of abnormal growth patterns. Stunted growth, distorted leaves or flowers, and the development of galls or tumors are all indications of plant diseases. These growth abnormalities can be the result of pathogens invading the plant's tissues and disrupting its normal growth processes.

Furthermore, students need to be observant of any visible signs of pests on plants as they can often be carriers of diseases. Look for insects, mites, or any other pests that may be feeding on the plants or causing physical damage. Some pests, such as aphids or whiteflies, can transmit viruses to the plants they infest, leading to further damage and disease development.

It is important to note that symptoms can vary depending on the type of plant and the specific disease at hand. Therefore, it is essential to have a basic understanding of the different types of plant diseases and their characteristic symptoms. Familiarize yourself with common plant pathogens, such as fungi, bacteria, viruses, and nematodes, and learn about the diseases they cause.

By recognizing the symptoms of plant diseases, students can take proactive measures to prevent and control them. Early detection is key to minimizing the spread and impact of diseases, which is why your role as a disease detective is so crucial. In the upcoming chapters, we will delve deeper into the world of plant pathology, exploring the causes, prevention, and management strategies for various plant diseases.

Remember, as a student of botany, your knowledge and skills can help protect plants and contribute to the overall health of our environment. So keep observing, learning, and unraveling the secrets of plant pathology as we embark on this journey together!

Leaf Symptoms

In the fascinating world of botany, we come across a wide range of plants that captivate us with their beauty and significance. However, just like humans, plants can fall victim to diseases and disorders that affect their growth and overall health. One of the key ways to identify these issues is by closely examining the symptoms that appear on the leaves.

Leaf symptoms provide valuable clues to diagnose and understand the health of a plant. By observing the changes in color, shape, texture, and overall appearance of the leaves, we can unravel the secrets of plant pathology and take necessary measures to restore their vitality.

Discoloration is one of the most common leaf symptoms. When leaves turn yellow, it often indicates a nutrient deficiency, such as lack of nitrogen. On the other hand, brown or black spots may be a sign of a fungal or bacterial infection. By learning to recognize these discolorations, students can play the role of disease detectives and take appropriate action to save the plants.

Leaf shape abnormalities are another important symptom to watch out for. Curling, wilting, or distorted leaves can indicate the presence of pests like aphids or mites, which suck the sap from the leaves, causing them to deform. Additionally, leaf edges that are serrated or have irregular patterns may signify a fungal infection or nutrient imbalance.

Texture changes in leaves should not be overlooked either. The presence of powdery mildew, a common fungal disease, can be identified by the powdery white substance that appears on the leaf surface. Conversely, a sticky or shiny residue may indicate an infestation of insects like aphids or scale insects.

Understanding leaf symptoms is crucial for botany students as it allows them to diagnose plant diseases accurately. Armed with knowledge and observation skills, students can take preventive measures, such as providing appropriate care, ensuring proper nutrition, and implementing pest control strategies.

In conclusion, leaf symptoms act as a key to unraveling the secrets of plant pathology. By closely observing and interpreting changes in leaf color, shape, and texture, students can become skilled disease detectives and successfully combat plant diseases. So, let us embark on this exciting journey of learning to identify leaf symptoms and protect the fascinating world of botany.

When it comes to diagnosing plant diseases, one of the key factors to look for is leaf symptoms. Just like humans, plants can also display visible signs of illness, and understanding these symptoms is crucial for botanists and plant pathologists. In this subchapter, we will explore the various leaf symptoms that can help students identify and unravel the secrets of plant pathology.

Leaf symptoms are the physical changes that occur in leaves when a plant is infected with a disease-causing agent, such as a bacterium, fungus, or virus. These symptoms can vary greatly depending on the type of pathogen involved and the specific plant species affected. By closely examining these symptoms, students can begin to unravel the mysteries of plant diseases and develop effective strategies for their prevention and control.

One common leaf symptom is chlorosis, which refers to the yellowing of leaves. Chlorosis can be caused by a variety of factors, including nutrient deficiencies, root damage, or infections. By carefully observing the pattern and intensity of chlorotic leaves, students can gain valuable insights into the underlying cause of the problem.

Another leaf symptom to watch out for is necrosis, which is the death of plant tissue. Necrotic leaf spots or blotches can be caused by pathogens invading the leaves and causing cell death. By examining the shape, size, and color of these spots, students can start to narrow down the potential culprits responsible for the disease.

Students should also pay attention to leaf wilting, a symptom often associated with water-related issues. Wilting can indicate a lack of water supply to the leaves, root damage, or infections that disrupt the plant's vascular system. By observing the timing and extent of wilting, students can gather valuable clues about the cause of the plant's distress.

Leaf symptoms can be further classified into specific types, such as leaf curling, leaf distortion, or leaf mottling. Each type of symptom may be indicative of different pathogens or environmental stressors. By learning to recognize and interpret these symptoms, students can become proficient disease detectives, able to identify the culprits behind plant diseases and devise appropriate treatments.

In conclusion, leaf symptoms are vital clues in the world of plant pathology. By understanding and interpreting these symptoms, students can unlock the secrets of plant diseases and contribute to the field of botany. So, keep your eyes peeled for chlorosis, necrosis, wilting, and other leaf symptoms, and embark on your journey as a disease detective today!

Stem Symptoms

When it comes to plant pathology, understanding the symptoms is crucial in diagnosing plant diseases. The stem of a plant is an essential part of its structure and plays a vital role in transporting nutrients and water throughout the plant. However, just like any other part of a plant, the stem is susceptible to various diseases that can hinder its proper functioning. In this subchapter, we will explore the symptoms of stem diseases and how to identify them.

One common symptom of stem diseases is discoloration. The stem may turn yellow, brown, or even black, depending on the specific disease. Discoloration can occur in patches or cover the entire stem, indicating the severity of the infection. It is important to note that discoloration can also be caused by other factors such as nutrient deficiencies, so it is crucial to consider other symptoms as well.

Another symptom to look out for is wilting. If the stem is infected, it may fail to transport water efficiently, leading to wilting of the leaves and overall drooping appearance of the plant. Wilting can occur gradually or suddenly, depending on the disease and its progression. It is important to differentiate between wilting caused by stem diseases and those caused by other factors such as lack of water or excessive heat.

In some cases, stem diseases can cause the stem to develop lesions or cankers. Lesions are areas of dead tissue that appear as dark, sunken spots on the stem. Cankers, on the other hand, are larger and more severe, often resulting in the death of entire branches or even the entire plant. Lesions and cankers can vary in shape and size depending on the specific disease, and they can also produce ooze or sap.

Other symptoms of stem diseases include swelling, galls, and deformations. Swelling occurs when the stem becomes enlarged and distorted due to the presence of pathogens. Galls are abnormal growths on the stem caused by the reaction of the plant to the infection. Deformations can range from stunted growth to irregular shapes of the stem.

Identifying these symptoms is crucial in diagnosing and managing stem diseases. By understanding the symptoms and their underlying causes, botany students can effectively take action to prevent the spread of diseases and protect the health of plants. Remember, early detection is key in combating plant diseases, so always keep an eye out for any unusual symptoms on the stems of your plants.

When studying plant pathology, one of the key areas of focus is identifying and understanding the symptoms that occur in different parts of a plant. In this subchapter, we will be exploring stem symptoms, which can provide valuable clues about the health and condition of a plant.

The stem is a vital part of a plant's structure, serving as a conduit for water, nutrients, and sugars. It also provides support for leaves, flowers, and fruits. Therefore, any abnormalities or diseases affecting the stem can have a significant impact on the overall health and productivity of a plant.

One of the most common stem symptoms is wilting. Wilting occurs when the stem loses its turgor pressure, leading to a drooping or sagging appearance of the plant. This symptom can be caused by various factors, including water stress, nutrient deficiencies, or even pathogenic infections. Understanding the underlying cause of wilting is crucial for implementing effective treatment strategies.

Another stem symptom to look out for is discoloration. When a plant's stem starts to change color, it can indicate the presence of diseases such as bacterial or fungal infections. For instance, a dark brown or black discoloration might suggest the presence of stem rot, a common fungal disease that affects many plant species. It is important to note that discoloration alone is not always conclusive evidence of a disease, so further investigation and laboratory analysis may be required for an accurate diagnosis.

Galls and cankers are also significant stem symptoms. Galls are abnormal growths that form on the stem, often caused by insects or nematodes. These growths can disrupt the flow of water and nutrients, leading to stunted growth and reduced vigor. Cankers, on the other hand, are localized dead areas on the stem caused by pathogens. They can weaken the stem, making it susceptible to breakage and further infections.

It is crucial for students studying botany to learn how to recognize and interpret stem symptoms accurately. By understanding these symptoms, students can become disease detectives, unraveling the secrets of plant pathology and helping to protect and preserve the health of our precious plant species.

In the upcoming chapters, we will delve deeper into specific stem diseases, their causes, and management strategies. Armed with this knowledge, students can become proactive in preventing and treating plant diseases, ensuring the sustainability and productivity of our botanical world.

Root Symptoms

When it comes to diagnosing plant diseases, it is crucial to pay attention to the symptoms exhibited by the roots. The roots are the foundation of a plant, responsible for anchoring it in the soil and absorbing nutrients and water. Therefore, any issues affecting the roots can have a significant impact on the overall health and survival of the plant.

One of the most common root symptoms is root rot. This occurs when the roots become infected with fungi, bacteria, or water molds, leading to their decay. As a result, the affected roots become soft, mushy, and discolored. Plants suffering from root rot often exhibit stunted growth, wilting, and yellowing of leaves. To prevent the spread of root rot, it is essential to ensure proper drainage, avoid overwatering, and practice good sanitation in the garden.

Another symptom to look out for is root galls. Galls are abnormal growths that form on the roots due to the presence of nematodes or bacteria. These galls can vary in size, shape, and color, depending on the pathogen responsible. Infected plants may show reduced vigor, yellowing leaves, and poor nutrient uptake. Crop rotation, planting resistant varieties, and using nematicides are some strategies to manage root galls effectively.

Root discoloration is another common symptom that can provide insights into the plant's health. Healthy roots are typically white or light-colored. However, when roots turn brown, black, or reddish, it may indicate various diseases or nutrient deficiencies. Brown roots, for example, can be a sign of root rot or lack of oxygen in the soil.

Blackened roots may indicate the presence of fungal pathogens, while reddish roots may suggest iron deficiency. Identifying the specific cause behind root discoloration is crucial for implementing appropriate treatment measures.

In conclusion, understanding and recognizing root symptoms are vital for diagnosing plant diseases accurately. By closely observing the roots, we can detect issues such as root rot, galls, and discoloration, which can provide valuable clues about the underlying problems affecting the plant's overall health. As budding botanists, it is essential to develop the skills to identify these symptoms and take appropriate action to ensure the well-being of plants in our care.

In the intricate world of plants, the root system serves as the foundation, providing essential support and nourishment. However, just like humans, plants can also fall victim to various diseases and infections that can greatly affect their overall health. As budding botanists, it is crucial to understand the root symptoms exhibited by plants, as they can be indicative of underlying problems.

One of the most common root symptoms is wilting. Wilting occurs when a plant's roots are unable to absorb sufficient water and nutrients from the soil. As a result, the leaves become limp, droopy, and often discolored. This is a clear indication that the plant is suffering from water stress, which can be caused by factors such as drought, root rot, or even overwatering.

Another prevalent root symptom is stunted growth. When a plant's roots are compromised by disease or pests, their ability to take up nutrients and establish a strong foundation is hindered. Consequently, the plant may exhibit slow or restricted growth, with undersized leaves and an overall diminutive stature. Stunted growth can be caused by various factors, including soil compaction, nutrient deficiencies, or the presence of harmful pathogens.

Root discoloration is yet another important symptom to look out for. Healthy roots typically have a white or light brown coloration. However, when plants are infected by pathogens, such as fungi or bacteria, the roots may exhibit discoloration, turning dark brown, black, or even red. Discolored roots indicate that the plant's defense mechanisms are being compromised, leaving it vulnerable to further damage.

Furthermore, root lesions are a common symptom associated with certain diseases. Lesions are essentially wounds or ulcers on the roots, caused by pathogens invading the plant's tissues. These lesions can vary in size and shape, and their presence suggests an ongoing battle between the plant and the invading pathogens.

As aspiring botanists, it is essential to be vigilant and observant when it comes to root symptoms. By recognizing and understanding these symptoms, we can diagnose and treat plant diseases more effectively. Proper identification and early intervention can help save plants from irreversible damage and ensure their continued growth and vitality. So, let's delve deeper into the fascinating world of plant pathology and unlock the secrets of the root symptoms that play a vital role in understanding and protecting the health of our beloved plants.

Flower and Fruit Symptoms

In the fascinating world of botany, flowers and fruits play a crucial role in the life cycle of plants. They are not only visually appealing but also serve as indicators of a plant's health. However, just like humans can fall ill, plants can also suffer from various diseases and infections. Recognizing the symptoms of these ailments is essential for students studying botany, as it allows them to become effective disease detectives in the field of plant pathology.

Flower symptoms are visible manifestations of diseases that affect the reproductive structures of plants. One common symptom is discoloration, where flowers may turn yellow, brown, or even black. This change in color could be a result of fungal or bacterial infections. Another symptom to watch out for is wilting, where flowers droop and lose their turgidity. This could be a sign of water-related issues or the presence of pathogens that block water movement within the plant.

Apart from discoloration and wilting, students should also be aware of deformities in flowers. These can range from misshapen petals to stunted growth. It is crucial to distinguish between natural variations in flower shapes and those caused by diseases. Additionally, abnormal growths, such as galls or tumors on flowers, can indicate the presence of pathogens or pests.

Moving on to fruit symptoms, students must learn to identify signs of diseases that affect the development and quality of fruits. One common symptom is rotting, where fruits become soft, discolored, and emit a foul odor. This can be caused by fungi or bacteria that thrive in moist conditions. Another symptom is premature ripening or fruit drop, where fruits ripen before reaching their full size or detach from the plant prematurely. Several factors, including pests, pathogens, or environmental stress, can contribute to this issue.

In the study of botany, being able to identify flower and fruit symptoms accurately is crucial for diagnosing and managing plant diseases effectively. By understanding these symptoms, students can develop essential skills to protect and preserve the health of plants. Whether it be in the field, laboratory, or greenhouse, disease detectives in the field of plant pathology play a vital role in ensuring the longevity and productivity of plants in our world. So, let's dive into the world of flower and fruit symptoms, and unravel the secrets of plant pathology together!

In the fascinating world of plant pathology, the study of flower and fruit symptoms plays a crucial role in understanding the health and well-being of plants. Flowers and fruits are not only beautiful and essential for reproduction in plants, but they are also vulnerable to various diseases and disorders. By recognizing and interpreting these symptoms, we can unravel the secrets of plant pathology and take appropriate measures to prevent the spread of diseases.

Flower symptoms can manifest in different ways, providing valuable clues about the underlying issues affecting plants. One common symptom is discoloration, where the petals may turn yellow, brown, or develop spots. This could indicate the presence of fungal or bacterial infections. Another symptom is wilting, where the flowers may droop or fail to open properly. Wilting could be caused by water stress, nutrient deficiencies, or even insect damage. Furthermore, deformities in the shape of flowers can be indicative of viral infections or genetic abnormalities. By closely observing these symptoms, we can identify the specific disease or disorder and take appropriate steps to mitigate its impact.

Fruit symptoms, on the other hand, are equally vital in diagnosing plant health. Many diseases affecting fruits are caused by pathogens that attack the plant's reproductive structures. For instance, rotting or decay of fruits is often caused by fungal infections that thrive in moist conditions. In addition, blemishes or scars on the fruit's surface can be a result of bacterial infections or physical damage. These symptoms not only affect the aesthetic appeal of fruits but may also render them unfit for consumption. By studying these symptoms, we can implement timely interventions to protect our crops and ensure a healthy harvest.

Understanding flower and fruit symptoms is of great significance to students interested in botany. By delving into the intricate details of these symptoms, we can gain insights into the complex interactions between plants and their environment. This knowledge equips us with the tools to become disease detectives, capable of identifying and solving plant health issues. Moreover, by studying these symptoms, we develop a deeper appreciation for the remarkable resilience and adaptability of plants in the face of challenges.

In conclusion, flower and fruit symptoms offer a fascinating window into the world of plant pathology. Recognizing and interpreting these symptoms enables us to diagnose and address diseases affecting plants. By studying these symptoms, students interested in botany can unlock the secrets of plant health and contribute to the field of plant pathology. Let us become disease detectives, unraveling the mysteries of flower and fruit symptoms and nurturing a healthier and more resilient plant kingdom.

Using Diagnostic Tools for Disease Identification

In the field of plant pathology, the ability to accurately identify diseases is of utmost importance. By understanding the cause and symptoms of plant diseases, scientists and botanists can develop effective strategies to control and manage them. One essential aspect of disease identification is the use of diagnostic tools, which enable researchers to pinpoint the pathogen responsible for the disease and devise appropriate treatment plans.

One commonly used diagnostic tool is the microscope. Through microscopic examination, scientists can study the morphology and structure of plant pathogens, such as fungi, bacteria, and viruses. By observing their unique characteristics, they can determine the specific pathogen causing the disease. Microscopy also aids in identifying the mode of infection and the extent of damage caused to the plant.

In addition to microscopy, molecular diagnostics have revolutionized disease identification in recent years. Techniques like polymerase chain reaction (PCR) and DNA sequencing allow scientists to detect and identify pathogens by analyzing their genetic material. This advanced tool has significantly improved the accuracy and speed of disease identification, enabling botanists to take prompt action to prevent further spread of diseases.

Another valuable diagnostic tool is serological testing. This method involves testing plant samples for the presence of specific antibodies or antigens associated with particular pathogens. By using techniques like enzyme-linked immunosorbent assay (ELISA), scientists can quickly detect the presence of pathogens, even in the absence of visible symptoms. Serological testing is particularly useful for detecting viral diseases, which often lack distinct visible symptoms.

Remote sensing technology is also becoming increasingly important in disease identification. By using satellite imagery and other remote sensing techniques, scientists can monitor changes in vegetation patterns and identify areas affected by diseases. This enables early detection and intervention, preventing the spread of diseases to neighboring plants.

In conclusion, the use of diagnostic tools in disease identification plays a crucial role in the field of plant pathology. Microscopy, molecular diagnostics, serological testing, and remote sensing technology are all valuable tools that enable scientists and botanists to accurately identify and manage plant diseases. By understanding the specific pathogens causing diseases, researchers can develop targeted and effective strategies to protect plant health and ensure sustainable agriculture.

In the fascinating world of plant pathology, the ability to accurately identify diseases is crucial for effective management and control. Just like detectives unraveling mysteries, disease detectives in the field of botany employ various diagnostic tools to identify and understand plant diseases. These tools enable them to make informed decisions and take appropriate measures to protect our precious plants.

One of the most commonly used diagnostic tools is visual observation. By carefully examining plant symptoms and signs, students can identify patterns and characteristics that are indicative of particular diseases. These symptoms may include discoloration, wilting, lesions, or abnormal growth patterns. For instance, a yellowing of leaves in a specific pattern may suggest a nutrient deficiency, while dark spots could indicate a fungal infection.

In addition to visual observation, disease detectives often rely on specialized equipment such as microscopes. Microscopic examination allows students to observe the intricate details of pathogens and their interactions with plant tissues. By studying the morphology of fungi, bacteria, or viruses, students can identify specific pathogens responsible for plant diseases.

Another vital diagnostic tool is the use of molecular techniques. These techniques involve analyzing the genetic material of pathogens to identify and differentiate between various species or strains. For instance, polymerase chain reaction (PCR) is a common molecular tool that amplifies specific DNA sequences for identification purposes. By comparing the DNA profiles of different pathogens, students can determine which one is responsible for a particular disease outbreak.

Furthermore, diagnostic kits and test strips are becoming increasingly popular among disease detectives. These kits provide rapid and on-site detection of pathogens by utilizing specific antibodies or enzymes that react with pathogen proteins or DNA. Students can easily use these kits to quickly identify diseases in the field, saving time and resources.

Lastly, students can also make use of online databases and resources to aid in disease identification. These platforms provide a wealth of information on various plant diseases, including symptoms, causal agents, and management strategies. By accessing these resources, students can enhance their knowledge and stay updated on the latest developments in the field of plant pathology.

In conclusion, using diagnostic tools is essential for disease identification in the field of botany. Visual observation, microscopes, molecular techniques, diagnostic kits, and online resources all contribute to accurate disease diagnosis. By mastering these tools, students can become skilled disease detectives, unraveling the secrets of plant pathology and preserving the health of our plant kingdom.

Microscopic Examination

In the fascinating world of plant pathology, the examination of samples under a microscope plays a crucial role in unraveling the secrets of diseases that affect plants. Microscopic examination is a powerful tool that allows us to dive deep into the microscopic world and explore the intricate details of plant pathogens and their effects on plants. In this subchapter, we will explore the importance of microscopic examination in the field of botany and how it aids disease detectives in their quest to understand and combat plant diseases.

Microscopic examination involves the use of a microscope, a device that magnifies small objects, to observe and analyze plant samples at a cellular level. By examining plant tissues, scientists can identify the presence of pathogens, observe their structures, and study the interaction between pathogens and plant cells. This helps in diagnosing the disease accurately and formulating effective strategies for disease management.

For students studying botany, microscopic examination offers a window into the intriguing world of plant diseases. By learning how to use a microscope and interpret the observations, students can develop a deeper understanding of the mechanisms behind plant diseases and their impact on plants. They can visualize the various structures of pathogens such as fungi, bacteria, and viruses, and comprehend how these microorganisms invade plants and cause diseases.

Microscopic examination also aids in the identification of plant pathogens. By observing the unique characteristics of different pathogens, students can learn to differentiate between different types of diseases and understand their specific symptoms. This knowledge is essential for effective disease management and prevention strategies.

Furthermore, microscopic examination allows students to explore the intricacies of plant defense mechanisms. By observing the interaction between pathogens and plant cells, students can gain insights into how plants respond to pathogenic attacks. They can study the structural and biochemical changes that occur in infected plants, helping them understand the ways in which plants defend themselves against diseases.

In conclusion, microscopic examination is a valuable tool in the field of botany, particularly in the study of plant pathology. It enables students to delve into the microscopic world of plant diseases, identify pathogens, understand disease symptoms, and analyze plant defense mechanisms. By mastering the art of microscopic examination, students can become skilled disease detectives, equipped with the knowledge and skills to unravel the secrets of plant pathology.

In the captivating world of plant pathology, one of the most crucial tools in unraveling the secrets of diseases is microscopic examination. This technique allows us to delve into the microscopic structures of plants and pathogens, providing invaluable insights into the intricate interactions between them. So, grab your magnifying lens and join us on this exciting journey of discovery!

Microscopic examination involves the use of a microscope to observe and analyze plant tissues, pathogen structures, and their interactions. This technique enables us to identify and understand the underlying causes of plant diseases, paving the way for effective management strategies. By examining the minute details of plant cells and pathogens, we can decipher the mechanisms of infection, the progression of diseases, and the impact they have on plant health.

To perform a microscopic examination, a small sample of the infected plant tissue is carefully collected and prepared for observation. Thin sections of the tissue are usually stained to highlight specific structures and enhance visibility. These stained sections are then placed under the microscope, where they unveil a hidden world teeming with life.

Under the lens, you will discover a plethora of fascinating structures. Plant cells, with their walls and organelles, will come into focus, displaying the intricate architecture that supports their vital functions. Meanwhile, pathogens such as fungi, bacteria, and viruses will reveal their own unique structures, which allow them to invade and colonize plant tissues.

Microscopic examination not only aids in disease diagnosis but also provides valuable insights into the epidemiology and life cycles of pathogens. By studying the spores, hyphae, and other reproductive structures of pathogens, we can unravel the mystery of how diseases spread and persist in the environment. This knowledge is crucial for developing strategies to prevent and manage plant diseases effectively.

As budding botanists and plant enthusiasts, understanding the microscopic world of plant pathology is an essential skill. Through microscopic examination, we can unlock the secrets of plant diseases and contribute to the development of sustainable and resilient agricultural practices. So, let's embark on this microscopic adventure and unravel the hidden secrets that lie beneath the surface of plants!

Serological Tests

In the field of plant pathology, serological tests play a vital role in diagnosing various plant diseases. These tests are based on the detection of specific antibodies or antigens in plant samples, helping researchers and plant pathologists identify the presence of pathogens accurately. By exploring the fascinating world of serological tests, students of botany can unravel the secrets of plant pathology and gain a deeper understanding of how diseases affect plants.

Serological tests are commonly used to detect viral, bacterial, and fungal pathogens in plants. These tests rely on the principle of antigen-antibody reactions, where antibodies specifically bind to antigens, leading to the formation of visible signals. The process begins with collecting plant samples from potentially infected plants. These samples are then processed to extract the target antigens or antibodies.

One of the widely used serological tests is the Enzyme-Linked Immunosorbent Assay (ELISA). ELISA utilizes the specific binding of antibodies to antigens to detect the presence of pathogens. In this test, plant samples are coated onto a surface, such as a microplate, and then treated with specific antibodies. If the plant sample contains the target pathogen, the antibodies will bind to the antigens, forming a complex. This complex can be visualized using an enzyme-linked secondary antibody, resulting in a color change or fluorescence that indicates the presence of the pathogen.

Another commonly employed serological test is the Western blot. This technique helps researchers detect specific proteins associated with plant pathogens. In a Western blot, plant proteins are separated using gel electrophoresis and transferred to a solid support, such as a membrane. The membrane is then treated with specific antibodies, which bind to the target proteins. By visualizing the bound antibodies, researchers can identify the presence of specific pathogens or disease-related proteins.

Serological tests provide students of botany with a powerful tool to investigate plant diseases and understand the mechanisms behind pathogen invasion. By utilizing these tests, researchers can accurately identify and diagnose plant diseases, enabling the development of effective strategies for disease management and prevention. As students delve into the world of serological tests, they will unlock the secrets of plant pathology and contribute to the field's ongoing efforts to protect and enhance the health of our plant ecosystems.

Serological tests play a crucial role in the field of plant pathology, allowing scientists to unravel the secrets behind various plant diseases. These tests utilize the principles of immunology to detect and identify specific pathogens in plants. For students interested in botany and plant pathology, understanding serological tests is essential for diagnosing and managing plant diseases effectively.

One of the most commonly used serological tests is the enzyme-linked immunosorbent assay (ELISA). ELISA is highly sensitive and can detect small amounts of pathogen proteins or antibodies present in plant tissues. This test involves the use of specific antibodies that bind to the target pathogen, indicating its presence. ELISA can help identify pathogens responsible for diseases like bacterial leaf spots, viral infections, or fungal diseases.

Another important serological test is the immunofluorescence assay (IFA). This technique uses fluorescent dyes that bind to specific antibodies, allowing scientists to visualize the presence of pathogens under a microscope. IFA is particularly useful for detecting viruses or bacteria in plant tissues, as the fluorescent signal provides clear evidence of their presence. This test helps researchers determine the extent of pathogen spread within plants and develop appropriate management strategies.

Students studying botany can also benefit from learning about the Western blot technique. Western blotting is a powerful tool for identifying and characterizing plant pathogens at the molecular level. It involves separating pathogen proteins using gel electrophoresis and then transferring them onto a membrane for detection using specific antibodies. This technique allows scientists to analyze the proteins produced by pathogens and gain insight into their structure and function.

Understanding serological tests is essential for students interested in plant pathology as it enables them to diagnose plant diseases accurately. By identifying the pathogens responsible for diseases, scientists can develop targeted strategies for disease management. This knowledge is crucial for ensuring the health and productivity of plants, which is vital for agriculture, horticulture, and environmental conservation.

In conclusion, serological tests are powerful diagnostic tools in the field of plant pathology. Students with an interest in botany can greatly benefit from understanding and utilizing these tests to identify and manage plant diseases. By mastering serological techniques like

ELISA, IFA, and Western blotting, students can become effective disease detectives, contributing to the health and well-being of plants worldwide.

Molecular Techniques

In the ever-evolving field of plant pathology, scientists have made groundbreaking discoveries using molecular techniques. These techniques enable researchers to study the genetic makeup of plants and the microorganisms that cause diseases, providing essential insights into plant health and disease management. In this subchapter, we will explore some of the key molecular techniques employed by disease detectives in the field of botany.

One of the most widely used techniques is DNA sequencing. DNA, or deoxyribonucleic acid, carries the genetic information of living organisms. By sequencing the DNA of plants and pathogens, scientists can identify specific genes that play a role in disease resistance or susceptibility. This information helps breeders develop resistant plant varieties and allows researchers to understand how diseases spread and evolve.

Another powerful tool in the molecular arsenal is polymerase chain reaction (PCR). PCR allows scientists to amplify specific regions of DNA, making it easier to detect pathogens in plant tissues. By targeting unique DNA sequences in the pathogen's genome, researchers can quickly and accurately identify the presence of harmful microorganisms. PCR has revolutionized disease diagnosis, speeding up the process and improving accuracy compared to traditional methods.

Genetic modification, or genetic engineering, is yet another molecular technique with tremendous potential in plant pathology. By introducing foreign genes into plant genomes, scientists can confer resistance to diseases that would otherwise devastate crops. This technique has led to the development of genetically modified organisms (GMOs) that are resistant to pests and diseases, thus reducing the need for chemical pesticides and enhancing food security.

Furthermore, molecular techniques are instrumental in studying the complex interactions between plants and pathogens. For instance, transcriptomics allows scientists to analyze the expression of genes in response to pathogen attack. This information helps identify key defense mechanisms activated by plants and how pathogens counteract them. Additionally, proteomics enables researchers to study the proteins produced during infection, shedding light on the molecular mechanisms underlying plant-pathogen interactions.

In conclusion, molecular techniques have revolutionized the field of plant pathology, enabling disease detectives to unravel the secrets of plant diseases. From DNA sequencing to PCR, these tools have provided invaluable insights into plant health, disease management, and the development of resistant plant varieties. As students of botany, understanding and harnessing these molecular techniques will empower you to contribute to the future of agriculture and ensure global food security.

In the world of botany and plant pathology, scientists and researchers rely on a variety of tools and techniques to unravel the secrets of plant diseases. One of the most powerful tools at their disposal is molecular techniques. These techniques have revolutionized the field by allowing scientists to study the genetic makeup of plants and the pathogens that infect them.

At its core, molecular techniques involve the manipulation and analysis of DNA and RNA molecules. By studying these molecules, scientists can gain insights into the underlying causes of plant diseases, identify specific pathogens, and develop strategies to combat them. Let's take a closer look at some of the key molecular techniques used in plant pathology.

DNA sequencing is a fundamental technique that allows scientists to determine the precise order of nucleotides in a DNA molecule. This information provides invaluable insights into the genetic makeup of plants and pathogens. By comparing the DNA sequences of different organisms, scientists can identify genes that may be responsible for disease resistance or susceptibility.

Polymerase Chain Reaction (PCR) is another essential molecular technique. PCR allows scientists to amplify specific regions of DNA, making it easier to study and analyze. This technique is particularly useful in identifying pathogens present in plant tissues. By targeting specific regions of the pathogen's DNA, scientists can determine whether it is present in a diseased plant and, if so, which specific pathogen is causing the disease.

Gel electrophoresis is a technique that separates DNA and RNA molecules based on their size and charge. This technique allows scientists to visualize and analyze the fragments of DNA or RNA generated through PCR or other molecular techniques. By examining the patterns of DNA or RNA fragments, scientists can gain insights into the genetic diversity of pathogens and trace their origins.

These are just a few examples of the molecular techniques used in plant pathology. Each technique has its strengths and limitations, but when used together, they provide a powerful toolbox for disease detectives. By harnessing the power of molecular techniques, scientists can better understand plant diseases and develop innovative solutions to protect our crops and ecosystems.

For students interested in botany and plant pathology, learning about molecular techniques is essential. These techniques are the backbone of modern plant pathology research and offer exciting opportunities for future scientific discoveries. Understanding the principles and applications of molecular techniques will not only enhance your knowledge but also empower you to contribute to the field and make a difference in the world of plant health.

Chapter 4: Causes and Transmission of Plant Diseases

Understanding Pathogens

In the fascinating world of botany, one cannot overlook the role of pathogens in shaping the health and well-being of plants. Pathogens are microscopic organisms that can cause diseases in plants, leading to devastating consequences for agricultural production and ecosystems. In this subchapter, we will delve into the intricacies of understanding pathogens, their types, and their impact on plants – an essential knowledge for all budding botanists.

To begin with, pathogens come in various forms, including viruses, bacteria, fungi, nematodes, and even parasitic plants. Each type of pathogen has its unique characteristics, modes of transmission, and effects on plants. Viruses, for instance, are tiny particles consisting of genetic material enclosed in a protein coat. They can hijack a plant's cellular machinery, causing a range of symptoms such as leaf discoloration, stunted growth, and even death. Bacteria, on the other hand, are single-celled organisms that can invade plant tissues, leading to wilt, rot, or cankers.

Fungi, another common group of pathogens, are multicellular organisms that thrive in damp environments. They can cause diseases such as powdery mildew, rust, or damping-off, which affect various parts of the plant, including leaves, stems, and roots. Nematodes, often referred to as microscopic worms, can also wreak havoc on plants by feeding on their roots, hindering nutrient uptake, and causing wilting or stunting. Lastly, parasitic plants like dodder and mistletoe establish a parasitic relationship with their host plants, siphoning off nutrients and weakening their hosts.

Understanding the life cycles and mechanisms of these pathogens is crucial for developing effective strategies to combat plant diseases. By studying their modes of transmission, such as through contact, insect vectors, or contaminated soil, botanists can devise preventive measures like crop rotation, quarantine, or the use of resistant plant varieties. Scientists also investigate the genetic makeup of pathogens to identify weak points that can be targeted through biological control methods or the development of disease-resistant plants using advanced breeding techniques.

As students of botany, it is paramount to comprehend the intricate interactions between plants and pathogens. Armed with this knowledge, we can contribute to the development of sustainable agricultural practices, ensure food security, and protect the biodiversity of our ecosystems. So, let us embark on this exciting journey of unraveling the secrets of plant pathology and become disease detectives, ready to tackle the challenges posed by pathogens and safeguard the health of our beloved plants.

Pathogens are microscopic organisms that can cause diseases in plants. In this subchapter, we will delve into the fascinating world of plant pathogens and explore how they affect the health and well-being of plants. By understanding these harmful organisms, we can better protect our beloved botanical friends and ensure a thriving plant kingdom.

What are Pathogens?
Pathogens are specialized microorganisms that invade plants, causing diseases that range from mild to severe. They come in various forms, including bacteria, fungi, viruses, and nematodes. Each type of pathogen has its unique characteristics and ways of infecting plants. By studying them, we can unravel their secrets and find effective strategies to combat plant diseases.

How do Pathogens Infect Plants?
Pathogens employ diverse strategies to infect plants and establish themselves within their hosts. Some pathogens enter plants through wounds or natural openings, such as stomata, while others penetrate directly through the plant's cell walls. Once inside, they multiply rapidly and disrupt the normal functioning of plant tissues, leading to disease symptoms.

Recognizing Disease Symptoms
Understanding the symptoms caused by pathogens is crucial for early detection and effective disease management. Symptoms may manifest as leaf spots, wilting, cankers, or stunted growth. By learning to recognize these signs, students can quickly identify and diagnose plant diseases, enabling prompt intervention.

Preventing and Managing Pathogen Infections
Prevention is always better than cure when it comes to plant diseases. By implementing good cultural practices, such as proper sanitation and crop rotation, students can minimize the risk of pathogen infections. Additionally, using resistant plant varieties, employing biological controls, and practicing integrated pest management can help combat pathogens effectively.

The   Role   of   Plant   Pathologists
Plant pathologists are scientists who study plant diseases caused by pathogens. They play a crucial role in identifying, characterizing, and managing plant pathogens. By conducting research and developing innovative strategies, plant pathologists contribute to the preservation of plant health and the sustainability of agriculture.

In conclusion, understanding pathogens is essential for students interested in botany. By comprehending the unique characteristics, infection strategies, and symptoms caused by plant pathogens, students can protect plants from diseases that can compromise their health and productivity. By becoming disease detectives, students can contribute to unraveling the secrets of plant pathology and ensuring a thriving plant kingdom for generations to come.

Fungal Pathogens

Fungi, a group of organisms that includes mushrooms and molds, can cause various diseases in plants. These fungal pathogens are responsible for significant damage to crops and plants in general, leading to decreased yields and economic losses. Understanding these fungal pathogens is crucial for students studying botany, as it helps them grasp the complexities of plant diseases and develop effective strategies to combat them.

Fungal pathogens can attack plants in several ways. Some fungi invade plant tissues directly, breaking down cell walls and causing rot or wilting. Others produce toxins that harm plants or interfere with their normal growth and development. Understanding the mechanisms by which these pathogens infect plants is essential for students to comprehend the disease cycle and how it can be interrupted.

One common example of a fungal pathogen is powdery mildew. This disease affects a wide range of plants, including roses, cucumbers, and grapes. Powdery mildew appears as a white powdery growth on the leaves, stems, and sometimes even the fruits of affected plants. Students studying botany need to understand the life cycle of powdery mildew, how it spreads, and the environmental conditions that favor its growth.

Another significant fungal pathogen is rust, which affects a variety of crops such as wheat, corn, and soybeans. Rust appears as reddish-brown pustules on the leaves, stems, and even the grains of infected plants. Students should learn about the life cycle of rust, including its dependence on alternate hosts, as well as the strategies employed by farmers to control its spread.

To effectively manage fungal pathogens, students must also be aware of cultural practices that can minimize disease incidence. These practices include crop rotation, sanitation, and proper plant spacing to create an unfavorable environment for fungal growth. Additionally, they need to understand the role of fungicides and biological control agents in disease management.

In conclusion, the study of fungal pathogens is crucial for students in the field of botany. By understanding the life cycles, modes of infection, and management strategies of these pathogens, students will be better equipped to tackle plant diseases and contribute to sustainable agriculture. Furthermore, this knowledge will empower them to develop innovative solutions to combat fungal pathogens and protect our valuable plant resources.

Fungi are a diverse group of organisms that play a crucial role in our ecosystem. However, some fungi can also cause diseases in plants, leading to significant losses in agriculture and forestry. Understanding these fungal pathogens is essential for students studying botany, as it provides insights into the complex world of plant diseases.

Fungal pathogens can infect various parts of a plant, including the roots, stems, leaves, and fruits. They can invade plant tissues through wounds, natural openings, or by penetrating the cell walls. Once inside the plant, they grow and reproduce, causing damage to the host. Common symptoms of fungal infections include wilting, discoloration, spotting, and decay.

One notorious fungal pathogen that students should be aware of is the powdery mildew. This pathogen affects a wide range of plants, including roses, cucumbers, and grapes. Powdery mildew appears as a white powdery substance on the surfaces of leaves and stems. As it spreads, the affected plant parts may become stunted, deformed, or even die. Students studying botany should learn about the life cycle of powdery mildew and the strategies to control its spread, such as pruning infected parts and applying fungicides.

Another important fungal pathogen is the rust fungus. Rusts are named for the characteristic reddish-brown spores that appear on infected plant parts. These spores can easily spread through wind or rain, causing widespread damage. Wheat rust, for example, can devastate entire fields of wheat, leading to significant losses in grain production. Students should explore the life cycle of rust fungi and the methods used to manage their impact, such as planting resistant cultivars and practicing crop rotation.

In addition to understanding the specific fungal pathogens, students studying botany should also learn about general principles of disease management. This includes cultural practices like maintaining proper plant nutrition, practicing good sanitation, and providing adequate air circulation. Integrated pest management, which combines multiple strategies, including biological controls and resistant cultivars, should also be emphasized.

By delving into the world of fungal pathogens, students gain valuable knowledge about the complex interactions between plants and their environment. This understanding will equip them with the tools to identify, manage, and prevent plant diseases, ultimately contributing to the sustainable cultivation of crops and the preservation of our natural ecosystems.

Bacterial Pathogens

In the world of plant pathology, a branch of botany that focuses on the study of plant diseases, bacterial pathogens play a crucial role in understanding the complexities of plant health. These microscopic organisms, commonly known as bacteria, can cause devastating diseases that affect the growth, development, and overall survival of plants.

Bacterial pathogens are unique in their ability to infiltrate plant tissues and establish an infection. They can enter plants through natural openings like stomata, which are small pores on the surface of leaves, or through wounds caused by insects, nematodes, or other environmental factors. Once inside the plant, they multiply rapidly, leading to the development of various symptoms.

One of the most well-known bacterial pathogens is Xylella fastidiosa, which causes a disease called Pierce's disease in grapevines. This pathogen blocks the xylem vessels, which are responsible for transporting water and nutrients throughout the plant, resulting in wilting, leaf scorch, and eventually death. Another notorious bacterial pathogen is Erwinia amylovora, the causative agent of fire blight in apple and pear trees. This pathogen attacks the blossoms, shoots, and fruits, causing them to turn black and giving the appearance of being scorched by fire.

Bacterial pathogens can also produce toxins that directly harm plants. For example, Pseudomonas syringae, a common pathogen in many crops, produces a toxin called syringomycin that damages plant cell membranes, leading to cell death. This can result in leaf spots, blighting, and necrosis, affecting the overall productivity and quality of the crop.

Controlling bacterial pathogens requires a combination of preventive measures and management strategies. Farmers and researchers employ cultural practices like crop rotation, use of disease-resistant varieties, and sanitation to minimize the risk of infection. In some cases, chemical treatments may be necessary, but their use should be judicious to avoid the development of resistant bacteria.

Understanding the world of bacterial pathogens is crucial for students studying botany and plant pathology. By unraveling the secrets of these microscopic organisms, students can contribute to the development of innovative solutions to combat plant diseases and ensure the health and productivity of our crops. Whether it is through research, fieldwork, or education, the study of bacterial pathogens is a fascinating and important field that holds great potential for the future of botany and plant health.

In the world of plant pathology, bacterial pathogens play a significant role in causing diseases in plants. These microscopic organisms can invade plants, reproduce rapidly, and damage their host's tissues, leading to devastating consequences for crops and natural ecosystems. In this subchapter, we will explore the fascinating world of bacterial pathogens and delve into their impact on plants.

Bacterial pathogens are different from fungi or viruses, as they are single-celled organisms without a true nucleus. They can be found in soil, water, and on plant surfaces, waiting for an opportunity to invade the host. Once inside, they exploit the plant's resources, causing a wide range of symptoms such as leaf spots, wilting, cankers, and even plant death.

One notorious example of a bacterial pathogen is Xylella fastidiosa, which causes devastating diseases in various crops, including citrus trees, grapevines, and olive trees. This bacterium colonizes the xylem vessels, blocking water and nutrient flow throughout the plant. As a result, the infected plants suffer from dehydration, leaf scorching, and eventual death. Understanding the mechanisms of bacterial pathogenesis like Xylella fastidiosa is crucial to develop effective control strategies and protect our agricultural systems.

To identify and manage bacterial pathogens, plant pathologists use a range of techniques. They employ advanced laboratory methods to isolate and identify the causative bacteria, as well as molecular tools to study their genetic makeup. Additionally, researchers investigate the interactions between bacteria and plants, studying how the host's immune system responds to infection. This knowledge helps in developing disease-resistant plant varieties and sustainable management practices.

As students interested in botany, understanding bacterial pathogens is essential as they have a significant impact on both agricultural and natural ecosystems. By unraveling the secrets of plant pathology, we can contribute to the development of sustainable farming practices, protect our environment, and ensure food security for future generations.

In the subsequent chapters, we will delve deeper into specific bacterial pathogens, their life cycles, and the strategies employed by scientists to combat these diseases. Get ready to embark on an exciting journey through the world of bacterial pathogens and unlock the secrets of plant pathology!

Viral Pathogens

In the vast field of plant pathology, one of the most intriguing and challenging areas of study is the understanding and control of viral pathogens. Viruses are microscopic infectious agents that can cause devastating diseases in plants, affecting their growth, development, and overall health. As budding disease detectives in the world of botany, it is essential for students to grasp the significance of viral pathogens and their impact on plant life.

Viral pathogens are unique in their structure and behavior. Unlike bacteria or fungi, viruses are not cells but rather strands of genetic material enclosed in a protein coat. They cannot reproduce or carry out metabolic processes on their own but instead rely on host cells to multiply. Once a virus enters a plant cell, it hijacks the cell's machinery and forces it to produce more viral particles, leading to the spread of the infection.

There are countless viral pathogens that infect plants, with each specialized to attack specific plant species or even certain parts of a plant. These pathogens can be transmitted through various means, including insect vectors, contaminated tools or equipment, infected seeds or plant material, and even from plant to plant through physical contact.

The consequences of viral infections on plants can be disastrous. Infected plants often display symptoms such as stunted growth, yellowing or mottled leaves, wilting, and distorted or deformed plant structures. These symptoms not only compromise the aesthetic appeal of plants but also affect their ability to carry out essential functions like photosynthesis, nutrient uptake, and reproduction.

To combat viral pathogens, it is crucial for students to understand the principles behind plant disease management. Prevention is the first line of defense, focusing on practices such as using disease-free seeds and plant material, maintaining proper sanitation in greenhouses or fields, and implementing quarantine measures to control the spread of infected plants.

When prevention fails, other strategies come into play. These strategies can include the use of resistant plant varieties, which are specifically bred to possess genetic traits that make them less susceptible to viral infections. Additionally, cultural practices like crop rotation, removal of infected plants, and pruning can help control the spread of viral pathogens and minimize their impact.

As students delve deeper into the world of plant pathology, understanding viral pathogens and their management becomes increasingly important. By unraveling the secrets of these microorganisms, students can contribute to the development of innovative techniques to protect our precious plants and ensure a healthier and more sustainable future for botany.

Understanding viral pathogens is crucial in the field of botany, as these microscopic organisms can have a significant impact on plant health and agriculture. In this subchapter, we will explore the world of viral pathogens, how they infect plants, and the strategies scientists employ to combat them.

Viral pathogens are viruses that infect plants, causing diseases that can result in stunted growth, reduced crop yields, and even death. These pathogens are not visible to the naked eye and can only be observed under powerful microscopes. Like human viruses, plant viruses cannot survive on their own and require a host to replicate and spread.

Plant viruses enter plants through various means, including insect vectors, contaminated soil, or infected seeds. Once inside the plant, viruses invade and hijack the plant's cellular machinery, forcing it to produce more virus particles. These particles then spread to other parts of the plant or to neighboring plants via insects, wind, or sap-feeding organisms.

Scientists employ several strategies to detect and combat viral pathogens. One common method is serological testing, which involves using specific antibodies to identify the presence of viral proteins in infected plants. This technique helps researchers determine the type of virus and its distribution within the plant.

Another approach is the use of molecular techniques such as polymerase chain reaction (PCR). By amplifying viral DNA or RNA, scientists can identify and characterize viral strains more accurately. This knowledge is crucial for developing effective control measures.

Prevention is an essential aspect of managing viral pathogens. Farmers and botanists implement strict sanitation practices, including the removal of infected plant material and the disinfection of tools and equipment. The use of resistant plant varieties and the employment of physical barriers, such as insect nets, can also help reduce viral spread.

In addition to prevention, scientists are continually working on developing new methods to control viral pathogens. This includes the use of genetic engineering to create plants with built-in resistance to specific viruses. By introducing genes that produce proteins that interfere with viral replication, researchers have successfully created crops that are less susceptible to viral infections.

Understanding viral pathogens and their impact on plants is crucial for botanists and students studying plant pathology. By staying informed about the latest research and developments in this field, students can become disease detectives who help unravel the secrets of plant health and contribute to finding sustainable solutions for agriculture.

Nematode Pathogens

Nematodes are microscopic worms that are found in abundance in soil and water. While most nematodes are harmless, some species can cause significant damage to plants, making them important pathogens in the field of plant pathology. In this subchapter, we will explore the fascinating world of nematode pathogens and their impact on plants.

Nematode pathogens, also known as plant-parasitic nematodes, are organisms that feed on plant roots or other plant parts, leading to stunted growth, wilting, and other symptoms of plant disease. They are capable of infecting a wide variety of plant species, including important crops such as potatoes, tomatoes, and soybeans. Understanding the biology and behavior of nematode pathogens is crucial for effective disease management strategies.

One of the most destructive nematode pathogens is the root-knot nematode. These tiny worms invade plant roots and induce the formation of swollen, knotted growths known as galls. The galls disrupt the normal functioning of the roots, resulting in reduced water and nutrient uptake by the plant. This can lead to stunted growth, yield loss, and even plant death. Root-knot nematodes are a major concern for farmers worldwide, and various control methods, including crop rotation and resistant plant varieties, are employed to manage their impact.

Another group of nematode pathogens is the cyst nematodes. These nematodes form cysts around their bodies, which protect them from harsh environmental conditions. Cyst nematodes can survive in the soil for many years and are particularly damaging to crops such as wheat, corn, and soybeans. Once hatched, the juvenile nematodes invade plant roots and establish feeding sites, causing nutrient depletion and reduced root function. Crop rotation, resistant varieties, and nematicides are some of the strategies used to control cyst nematodes.

In addition to root-knot and cyst nematodes, there are many other nematode pathogens that affect various plant species. The subchapter will provide an overview of these pathogens, including their life cycles, modes of infection, and the symptoms they cause in plants. It will also discuss the importance of nematode diagnostics and the role of plant pathologists in studying and managing nematode diseases.

Understanding the biology and impact of nematode pathogens is essential for students interested in botany and plant pathology. By unraveling the secrets of nematode pathogens, students can gain valuable insights into the intricate interactions between plants and their pathogens, ultimately contributing to the development of sustainable and effective disease management strategies in agriculture.

Nematodes, also known as roundworms, are microscopic organisms that play a significant role in plant pathology. These tiny creatures are found in various soil environments and can cause devastating diseases in plants. In this subchapter, we will explore the fascinating world of nematode pathogens and their impact on plant health.

Nematodes are incredibly diverse and can be found in almost every ecosystem on Earth. While most nematodes are harmless, some species have evolved to become parasitic, feeding on plant roots and causing significant damage. These parasitic nematodes can be classified into two main groups: sedentary and migratory.

Sedentary nematodes are known for their ability to establish a permanent feeding site within plant roots. They inject specialized substances into the plant cells, inducing the formation of a unique feeding structure called a syncytium. This feeding site provides the nematode with a constant supply of nutrients, causing stunted growth, yellowing leaves, and overall plant decline.

Migratory nematodes, on the other hand, move freely through the soil, feeding on plant roots as they travel. They cause damage by physically injuring the roots and creating entry points for other pathogens, such as bacteria and fungi, to invade. This combination of direct damage and secondary infections can lead to severe plant disease and even death.

Understanding nematode pathogens is crucial for botany students as it allows them to recognize and manage these diseases effectively. Diagnosis of nematode infections involves careful observation of plant symptoms, soil sampling, and laboratory analysis. Nematode control strategies include the use of resistant plant varieties, crop rotation, and the application of nematicides, which are chemical compounds specifically designed to target nematodes.

Botany students should also be aware of the importance of integrated pest management (IPM) techniques when dealing with nematode pathogens. IPM involves combining multiple control strategies to minimize the use of chemicals and promote sustainable plant health. This approach includes cultural practices such as proper irrigation, soil amendments, and biological control methods, such as the use of beneficial nematodes that prey on the harmful ones.

In conclusion, nematode pathogens pose a significant threat to plant health and productivity. As botany students, it is crucial to understand their biology, their impact on plants, and the various management strategies available. With this knowledge, we can work towards unraveling the secrets of nematode pathogenesis and contribute to the development of sustainable solutions for plant diseases.

Modes of Disease Transmission

Understanding how diseases are transmitted is crucial in the field of plant pathology. By identifying the modes of disease transmission, students of botany can gain valuable insights into the spread and control of plant diseases. This subchapter will explore the various ways in which diseases can be transmitted, providing students with a comprehensive understanding of disease dynamics in plants.

1. Direct Contact: Some diseases can be transmitted through direct contact between plants. This can occur through physical contact, such as when infected plant tissues touch healthy ones, or via root grafts between neighboring plants. Students will learn how to recognize the signs of direct contact transmission and understand the importance of isolating infected plants to prevent further spread.

2. Airborne Transmission: Many plant diseases are spread through the air. This can happen when infected plants release spores or other infectious particles into the atmosphere, which are then carried by wind currents to healthy plants. Students will discover the importance of wind patterns in disease transmission and learn how to identify diseases that are commonly spread through airborne means.

3. Soil-borne Transmission: Soil is a common reservoir for plant pathogens. In this section, students will explore how diseases can be transmitted through the soil, either by direct contact between roots or through the movement of contaminated soil particles. They will learn about the role of soil management practices in disease prevention and discover strategies for reducing soil-borne disease transmission.

4. Vector Transmission: Some plant diseases rely on vectors, such as insects or other animals, to spread from one plant to another. This section will introduce students to the concept of vector transmission and highlight the importance of understanding the biology and behavior of these vectors in disease control. Students will also learn about the various mechanisms by which vectors transmit diseases, such as feeding on infected plants or carrying infectious particles on their bodies.

5. Human-mediated Transmission: Humans can also play a role in disease transmission, whether unintentionally through agricultural practices or intentionally through the movement of infected plant materials. Students will explore the potential risks associated with human-mediated disease transmission and understand the importance of implementing biosecurity measures to prevent the spread of plant diseases.

By delving into the modes of disease transmission, students of botany will gain a deeper understanding of the complex dynamics underlying plant diseases. Armed with this knowledge, they will be better equipped to identify, prevent, and control plant diseases, ultimately contributing to the field of plant pathology and the health of our agricultural systems.

Understanding how diseases are transmitted is crucial in the field of botany. As aspiring botanists, it is important to unravel the secrets of disease transmission to effectively combat plant pathogens and protect our precious plant species. In this subchapter, we will explore the various modes of disease transmission in plants.

1. Direct Contact: One of the most common modes of disease transmission is through direct contact. This occurs when a healthy plant comes into contact with an infected plant or its contaminated parts. It could be through physical contact between plants, or through the use of contaminated tools, equipment, or hands during gardening or agricultural practices. It is essential to practice proper sanitation and hygiene to prevent the spread of diseases through direct contact.

2. Airborne Transmission: Many plant diseases are spread through the air. Fungal spores, bacteria, and viruses can be carried by wind currents over long distances and infect healthy plants. This mode of transmission is particularly challenging to control, as pathogens can travel far and wide. Understanding wind patterns and implementing preventive measures such as crop rotation, proper spacing between plants, and the use of windbreaks can help reduce the risk of airborne disease transmission.

3. Waterborne Transmission: Water plays a significant role in the spread of plant diseases. Pathogens can be present in irrigation water, rainfall, or standing water, and can infect plants through their roots, leaves, or fruits. Waterborne diseases are particularly common in humid and rainy regions. Proper water management, including the use of clean water sources and well-draining soil, can help minimize the risk of waterborne disease transmission.

4. Vector Transmission: Some diseases rely on vectors, such as insects, nematodes, or other organisms, to spread from one plant to another. These vectors act as carriers, transmitting the pathogens as they feed on plants. Examples include aphids spreading plant viruses or nematodes transmitting soil-borne diseases. Controlling vector

populations, using insecticides or biological controls, can help reduce the spread of diseases through vector transmission.

5. Seed Transmission: Another important mode of disease transmission is through infected seeds. Pathogens can survive inside seeds and germinate along with the plant, causing disease in the new generation. Seed treatments, such as hot water treatment or chemical treatments, can help eliminate pathogens from seeds and reduce the risk of seed transmission.

Understanding these modes of disease transmission is crucial for effective disease management in botany. By implementing preventive measures and adopting best practices, we can minimize the impact of plant diseases and ensure the health and vitality of our plant species. Remember, as disease detectives, it is our responsibility to unravel these secrets and protect our botanical world.

Soil-Borne Diseases

Introduction: Unraveling the Secrets of Soil-Borne Diseases

Welcome to the fascinating world of plant pathology, where we uncover the mysteries and secrets behind plant diseases. In this subchapter, we will delve into the realm of soil-borne diseases, a significant aspect of plant health. Understanding soil-borne diseases is crucial for students interested in botany, as it provides valuable knowledge about the intricate relationship between plants and their environment.

Exploring the Underworld: What are Soil-Borne Diseases?

Soil-borne diseases refer to the group of plant infections caused by pathogens lurking in the soil. These pathogens can include fungi, bacteria, viruses, and nematodes, which target various parts of the plant, including the roots and stem. As students passionate about botany, it is essential to comprehend how these organisms affect plant health and how we can manage them.

Common Soil-Borne Diseases: Identifying the Culprits

In this section, we will discuss some well-known soil-borne diseases that students studying botany should be familiar with. For instance, damping off, caused by certain fungi, leads to the rotting of young seedlings, hindering their growth. Another disease, Fusarium wilt, caused by a soil-borne fungus, affects a wide range of plants by blocking the vascular system, resulting in wilting and death.

Understanding Disease Management: Prevention and Control

As aspiring botanists, it is crucial to learn about disease management strategies. Prevention is always better than cure, and in the case of soil-borne diseases, it involves implementing good sanitation practices, crop rotation, and the use of disease-resistant plant varieties. Additionally, incorporating organic matter into the soil can enhance its health and suppress the development of soil-borne pathogens.

The Role of Soil Health: Nurturing Disease-Free Plants

Healthy soil is the foundation for healthy plants. In this section, we will discuss the importance of maintaining soil health to prevent soil-borne diseases. Students will learn about the significance of pH levels, nutrient availability, and soil structure in promoting plant vigor and resilience against pathogens.

Conclusion: The Never-Ending Quest for Plant Health

In the world of plant pathology, the battle against soil-borne diseases is ongoing. However, armed with knowledge and a passion for botany, students can play a crucial role in unraveling the secrets of these diseases. By understanding the causes, identifying the symptoms, and implementing effective management strategies, students will become disease detectives, actively contributing to the well-being of our beloved plants. So, let us embark on this exciting journey and continue to explore the intricate relationship between plants and their pathogens.

In the fascinating world of plant pathology, scientists are like detectives, unraveling the secrets behind diseases that affect plants. One significant area of investigation is soil-borne diseases, which pose a threat to the health and productivity of plants. In this subchapter, we will explore the mysteries of soil-borne diseases and their impact on plants.

Soil-borne diseases are caused by pathogens that reside in the soil, waiting for an opportunity to infect susceptible plants. These pathogens include fungi, bacteria, viruses, and nematodes. They can attack various parts of the plant, such as the roots, stems, leaves, or even the entire plant. Understanding these diseases is crucial for botanists, as it helps them develop strategies to prevent and manage them effectively.

One common soil-borne disease is Fusarium wilt, caused by the fungus Fusarium oxysporum. This pathogen invades the plants' vascular system, blocking the flow of water and nutrients. As a result, plants wilt, turn yellow or brown, and eventually die. Another notable disease is crown gall, caused by the bacterium Agrobacterium tumefaciens. It forms tumors on the plant's roots or stems, disrupting the normal growth and development.

Nematodes, microscopic worms, are also responsible for soil-borne diseases. Root-knot nematodes are particularly notorious. They invade the roots, causing the formation of characteristic galls that hinder the plant's ability to absorb water and nutrients. This leads to stunted growth, reduced yield, and sometimes death.

Preventing soil-borne diseases requires a multifaceted approach. Crop rotation is a common practice that involves growing different plant species in sequence to disrupt the lifecycle of pathogens. Soil solarization, where the soil is covered with a transparent plastic sheet to trap heat, can also be effective in killing pathogens. Additionally, planting disease-resistant varieties and maintaining good soil health through practices like composting and proper irrigation can help reduce the risk of infections.

To diagnose and manage soil-borne diseases, botanists employ various techniques. They conduct soil tests and microscopic examinations to identify the pathogens present. They also use cultural practices, such as removing infected plants and sanitizing tools, to prevent the spread of diseases. In some cases, chemical treatments may be necessary, but they are usually employed as a last resort.

By studying soil-borne diseases, botanists can unravel the secrets behind these hidden threats to plants' health. Armed with this knowledge, they can develop strategies to protect our crops and ensure food security. As students of botany, understanding soil-borne diseases and their management is essential for becoming future disease detectives and safeguarding the world's plants.

Airborne Diseases

Airborne diseases are a fascinating aspect of plant pathology that students studying botany should be aware of. These diseases are caused by pathogens that are transmitted through the air, making them highly contagious and easily spread. In this subchapter, we will delve into the world of airborne diseases, exploring their causes, transmission methods, and the impact they have on plants.

One of the most common airborne diseases in plants is powdery mildew. This disease is caused by a fungus that thrives in humid conditions and forms a white, powdery substance on the leaves, stems, and flowers of infected plants. It spreads through the air, making it highly contagious and capable of affecting a wide range of plant species. Students will learn about the lifecycle of powdery mildew and the various control methods that can be employed to prevent its spread.

Another notable airborne disease is rust. Rust is caused by fungal pathogens that produce spores, which are easily carried by the wind. This disease manifests as orange or brownish-colored pustules on the leaves, stems, and fruits of infected plants. It can have devastating effects on crops and is a significant concern for farmers and botanists alike. Students will explore the life cycle of rust pathogens, the conditions favorable for their growth, and the strategies employed to manage and control rust outbreaks.

Students will also gain insight into the importance of understanding airborne diseases in the context of plant pathology. By studying these diseases, students will learn how to identify and diagnose them, understand their impact on plant health, and develop effective control measures. They will also explore the role of environmental factors, such as humidity and temperature, in the transmission and development of airborne diseases.

In conclusion, the study of airborne diseases is crucial for students interested in botany. By understanding the causes, transmission methods, and impact of these diseases, students can become proficient disease detectives, capable of unraveling the secrets of plant pathology. This knowledge will enable them to protect and preserve plant health, contributing to the field of botany and ensuring the sustainability of our ecosystems.

In the vast world of plant pathology, there is a fascinating and often overlooked aspect that affects both plants and humans: airborne diseases. These diseases are caused by pathogens that travel through the air and can infect plants, causing devastating damage to crops, gardens, and natural ecosystems. Understanding airborne diseases is crucial for students interested in botany, as it sheds light on the complex interactions between plants and their environment.

Airborne diseases are primarily caused by microorganisms such as fungi, bacteria, and viruses. These pathogens are tiny and lightweight, allowing them to become airborne and travel with ease. Once in the air, they can be carried by wind currents over long distances, spreading rapidly and infecting susceptible plants.

One of the most well-known airborne diseases is powdery mildew, a fungal infection that affects a wide range of plants. This disease manifests as a powdery white or gray coating on the leaves, stems, and flowers of infected plants. Powdery mildew can stunt plant growth, reduce yield, and even lead to plant death if left untreated.

Another notorious airborne disease is bacterial leaf spot, which affects various plant species. It is characterized by dark, water-soaked lesions on the leaves, causing them to wither and die. Bacterial leaf spot can be particularly devastating in agricultural settings, as it can rapidly spread through a field, leading to significant yield losses.

Viruses also play a significant role in airborne diseases. Plant viruses are often transmitted by insects such as aphids or whiteflies, but they can also become airborne through infected plant debris or pollen. Once a virus enters a plant, it can disrupt its normal growth and development, leading to stunted growth, yellowing of leaves, and other visible symptoms.

Preventing and managing airborne diseases requires a combination of proactive measures. Crop rotation, which involves planting different crops in a specific sequence, can help break the disease cycle and reduce the buildup of pathogens in the soil. Additionally, practicing good sanitation, such as removing infected plant debris and weeds, can help minimize the spread of airborne diseases.

For students interested in botany, studying airborne diseases provides valuable insights into the delicate balance between plants and their environment. By understanding the mechanisms of airborne disease transmission and the impact they have on plants, students can contribute to finding sustainable solutions for managing these pathogens and protecting our crops and natural ecosystems.

In conclusion, airborne diseases are a captivating and critical aspect of plant pathology. Students interested in botany should delve into the study of these diseases to gain a deeper understanding of how pathogens can travel through the air and impact plants. By unraveling the secrets of airborne diseases, students can contribute to the field of plant pathology and work towards safeguarding our botanical world.

Vector-Borne Diseases

In the vast realm of plant pathology, one cannot overlook the role of vector-borne diseases. These diseases are caused by pathogens that are transmitted from one host to another through the intervention of vectors. A vector can be any living organism, such as insects, mites, nematodes, or even birds, that carries and spreads the pathogen. Vector-borne diseases pose a significant threat to plants, affecting not only their health but also the overall agricultural productivity.

Understanding the dynamics of vector-borne diseases is essential for students studying botany and interested in plant pathology. By unraveling the secrets behind these diseases, we can develop effective strategies to combat and control them, thus protecting our plants and ensuring food security.

Insects, with their ability to fly and crawl, are the most common vectors of plant diseases. Aphids, for instance, are notorious for transmitting viruses to a variety of crops, including vegetables, fruits, and ornamental plants. These tiny pests pierce the plant's tissues, injecting the virus into the cells, and then move on to the next plant, spreading the infection. Similarly, leafhoppers, whiteflies, and beetles play significant roles in spreading diseases like bacterial wilt, yellowing diseases, and fungal infections.

Mites, on the other hand, are microscopic pests that inhabit the undersides of leaves. They can transmit pathogens like viruses and fungi to plants, causing diseases like powdery mildew and rust. These diseases can severely impact the plant's ability to photosynthesize, leading to stunted growth and reduced yield.

Nematodes, often referred to as soil-dwelling worms, can also act as vectors for plant diseases. These microscopic organisms invade the plant's roots, causing root galls and disrupting nutrient uptake. They can transmit viruses, bacteria, and fungi, leading to diseases such as root-knot nematode disease and ring rot.

Birds, although not commonly associated with vectors, can also play a role in spreading plant diseases. They can unknowingly carry fungal spores on their feathers or beaks, transferring them from one plant to another. This can result in diseases like bird's eye spot, affecting fruits and leaves.

To effectively manage vector-borne diseases, it is crucial to identify the vectors responsible for transmitting specific pathogens. This knowledge allows scientists and plant pathologists to develop targeted control measures. These may include the use of insecticides, crop rotation, biological control agents, or breeding resistant plant varieties.

As students delving into the fascinating world of botany, understanding the complexities of vector-borne diseases is vital. By acquiring knowledge about these diseases and their vectors, you will be better equipped to contribute to the development of sustainable and effective strategies for disease management, safeguarding the health and productivity of our beloved plants.

Vector-Borne Diseases are a fascinating and important area of study within the field of plant pathology. In this subchapter, we will explore the intricate relationship between plants, pathogens, and the vectors that transmit diseases to them. This knowledge is crucial for students interested in botany, as it provides a deeper understanding of the complex dynamics that can affect plant health.

Vector-borne diseases are caused by pathogens that are transmitted by various organisms, known as vectors. These vectors can include insects, such as aphids and beetles, as well as mites, nematodes, and even birds and mammals. These organisms play a vital role in the spread of diseases, acting as carriers or reservoirs for pathogens.

One of the most well-known vector-borne diseases in plants is the citrus greening disease, caused by a bacterium called Candidatus Liberibacter asiaticus. This disease is primarily transmitted by the Asian citrus psyllid, a tiny insect that feeds on citrus trees. By understanding the life cycle of the psyllid and its relationship with the bacterium, researchers can develop strategies to control the spread of the disease and protect citrus crops.

Another example is the spread of tomato spotted wilt virus, which is transmitted by thrips, small insects that feed on plants. The virus can cause devastating damage to tomato and other vegetable crops. By studying the behavior and biology of thrips, scientists can devise methods to minimize the transmission of the virus and protect susceptible plants.

Understanding vector-borne diseases is crucial for plant pathologists and botanists because these diseases can have significant economic and ecological consequences. Outbreaks can lead to crop losses, impacting food security and livelihoods. Additionally, the introduction of invasive vectors can disrupt ecosystems and affect biodiversity.

By learning about vector-borne diseases, students can develop a deeper appreciation for the complexity of plant-pathogen interactions. They can also contribute to the development of sustainable and effective strategies to manage these diseases, such as the use of biocontrol agents or breeding resistant plant varieties.

In conclusion, vector-borne diseases play a significant role in plant pathology and have a direct impact on botany. By unraveling the secrets of these diseases, students can gain valuable insights into the intricate relationships between plants, pathogens, and vectors. This knowledge will not only expand their understanding of plant health but also empower them to contribute to the field of plant pathology and the development of innovative solutions to combat vector-borne diseases.

Seed and Plant Material Transmission

Introduction:

In the world of botany, the transmission of diseases through seed and plant material is a vital topic to understand. Plants can be affected by various pathogens, including bacteria, fungi, viruses, and nematodes. These pathogens can cause severe damage to crops and gardens, leading to reduced yields and economic losses. In this subchapter, we will delve into the fascinating world of seed and plant material transmission, exploring how diseases can spread and what measures can be taken to prevent their transmission.

Understanding Seed Transmission:

Seeds are the starting point for most plants, making them a crucial factor in disease transmission. Some pathogens can infect the embryo inside the seed, leading to diseased plants from the moment they germinate. This type of transmission is called seedborne transmission. Other pathogens may reside on the seed surface or within the seed coat, leading to contamination of the soil or subsequent generations of plants.

Preventing Seed Transmission:

To prevent the transmission of diseases through seeds, it is important to ensure that only healthy seeds are used for planting. This can be achieved through seed treatments, such as hot water treatments or chemical treatments, which eliminate or reduce the pathogens present on the seed surface. Additionally, proper storage conditions should be maintained to prevent the growth of pathogens within the seeds.

Plant Material Transmission:

Apart from seeds, diseases can also be transmitted through vegetative plant parts, such as cuttings, bulbs, and tubers. These plant materials may carry pathogens from one location to another, spreading diseases to new areas. It is crucial to inspect and quarantine plant materials before introducing them to new environments to prevent disease outbreaks.

Preventing Plant Material Transmission:

To prevent the transmission of diseases through plant materials, it is important to source them from reputable suppliers. Quarantine measures should be implemented to inspect and monitor incoming plant materials for any signs of disease. Additionally, proper sanitation practices should be followed, such as sterilizing tools and equipment used for plant propagation.

Conclusion:

Understanding the transmission of diseases through seed and plant materials is essential for students studying botany. By learning about the various ways pathogens can spread, students can take proactive measures to prevent disease outbreaks and protect crops and gardens. Through proper seed treatment, careful inspection of plant materials, and adherence to sanitation practices, students can become disease detectives in the field of botany, ensuring the health and productivity of plants for years to come.

In the fascinating world of botany, the transmission of disease-causing agents through seed and plant material is a crucial aspect that students must understand. This subchapter will delve into the intriguing process of how diseases can be transmitted through seeds and other plant materials. By unraveling these secrets of plant pathology, students will gain a deeper understanding of the importance of disease prevention and management in the field of botany.

When it comes to seed transmission, it is essential to recognize that seeds can carry diseases in two ways: externally and internally. Externally transmitted diseases are those that reside on the outer surface of the seed, while internally transmitted diseases are those that penetrate the seed coat and reside within the seed itself. Understanding the difference between these two modes of transmission is key to developing effective disease control strategies.

Seed transmission can occur through various means, including direct contact with infected seeds, contaminated soil, or even through insect vectors. It is crucial for students to learn about the different pathogens that can be transmitted through seeds, such as bacteria, fungi, and viruses, and how they can affect plant health.

Apart from seeds, plant materials like cuttings, bulbs, tubers, and rhizomes can also serve as vehicles for disease transmission. These plant parts can harbor pathogens and spread diseases when used for propagation or planting. Students must understand the importance of using disease-free plant materials to prevent the introduction and spread of diseases in new areas.

Preventing and managing seed and plant material transmission is vital for maintaining healthy crops and natural ecosystems. Students will learn about various disease prevention measures, such as seed treatment, heat treatment, and disease testing, which can help eliminate or reduce the transmission of pathogens through seeds and plant materials.

Moreover, students will be introduced to the concept of quarantine and how it plays a crucial role in preventing the introduction and spread of diseases through seed and plant material movement across different regions and countries. They will understand the significance of adhering to quarantine regulations and the potential consequences of not doing so.

By understanding the mechanisms and implications of seed and plant material transmission, students will be equipped with the knowledge needed to ensure the health and productivity of plants in various botanical settings. This subchapter will not only enhance their understanding of botany but also instill a sense of responsibility in disease prevention and management in the field of plant pathology.

Chapter 5: Prevention and Control of Plant Diseases

Cultural Practices for Disease Prevention

In the world of botany, diseases can wreak havoc on plants, leading to reduced yields, stunted growth, and even death. However, there are several cultural practices that students can adopt to prevent and manage plant diseases effectively. By understanding and implementing these practices, students can become disease detectives, unraveling the secrets of plant pathology and ensuring the health and vitality of their botanical specimens.

One of the most crucial cultural practices for disease prevention is crop rotation. This technique involves planting different plant species in a specific order or sequence, ensuring that the same plant family is not grown in the same location year after year. Crop rotation helps break the life cycle of pathogens that rely on host-specific plants, reducing the risk of disease outbreaks. By rotating crops, students can prevent the buildup of pathogens in the soil and maintain the overall health of their plants.

Another important practice is sanitation. Students should keep their gardening tools, pots, and other equipment clean and free from disease-causing organisms. Regularly disinfecting tools and containers can prevent the transmission of pathogens from one plant to another. Additionally, removing and disposing of infected plant debris promptly can help eliminate potential sources of infection.

Proper plant spacing is also essential for disease prevention. When plants are crowded, there is limited airflow, which creates a favorable environment for fungal diseases. By providing adequate spacing between plants, students can promote air circulation, reducing the likelihood of disease development.

Furthermore, watering practices play a significant role in disease prevention. Overwatering can create conditions that favor the growth of pathogens, so it is important for students to water their plants judiciously. Watering in the morning allows plants to dry off during the day, minimizing the risk of diseases caused by prolonged leaf wetness.

Lastly, students should select disease-resistant plant varieties whenever possible. Plant breeders have developed cultivars that exhibit natural resistance to specific diseases. By choosing resistant varieties, students can reduce the likelihood of disease outbreaks and minimize the need for chemical treatments.

In conclusion, cultural practices for disease prevention are vital in the field of botany. Crop rotation, sanitation, proper plant spacing, appropriate watering, and selecting disease-resistant plant varieties are all effective strategies for ensuring the health and vitality of plants. By implementing these practices, students can become disease detectives, unraveling the secrets of plant pathology and contributing to the field of botany.

In the world of botany, understanding and implementing cultural practices for disease prevention is essential for maintaining healthy plants and preventing the spread of plant pathogens. By adopting and following these practices, students can become disease detectives and unravel the secrets of plant pathology.

One of the fundamental cultural practices for disease prevention is crop rotation. This practice involves changing the plant species grown in a particular area each season or year. By rotating crops, students can disrupt the life cycles of pathogens that may have built up in the soil. Different plant species have varying susceptibility to certain diseases, and rotating crops helps break the cycle of infection, reducing the risk of disease outbreaks.

Another important practice is the removal and destruction of infected plant material. Students should be vigilant in observing plants for any signs of disease, such as wilting, discoloration, or abnormal growth. If any plants are found to be infected, they should be promptly removed and destroyed to prevent the spread of pathogens to healthy plants nearby. It is crucial to properly dispose of infected plant material, as some pathogens can survive outside the host and continue to infect other plants.

Maintaining good sanitation practices is also vital for disease prevention. Students should regularly clean and disinfect their gardening tools and equipment to prevent the transmission of pathogens. Additionally, they should practice good hygiene, such as washing their hands thoroughly before and after working with plants, to minimize the risk of spreading diseases.

Proper irrigation practices can also help prevent diseases in plants. Overwatering can create a favorable environment for pathogens to thrive, so students should aim for a balanced and appropriate watering regimen. It is important to water plants at their base and avoid wetting the leaves, as this can promote the growth of foliar diseases.

Lastly, promoting biodiversity in the garden can contribute to disease prevention. By planting a variety of plant species, students can reduce the risk of widespread outbreaks caused by specific pathogens. Different plants attract different pests and diseases, and a diverse garden can disrupt the life cycles of pests and limit their impact on crops.

In conclusion, understanding and implementing cultural practices for disease prevention is crucial for students interested in botany. By adopting practices such as crop rotation, removal of infected plant material, good sanitation, proper irrigation, and promoting biodiversity, students can protect their plants and unravel the secrets of plant pathology as disease detectives.

Crop Rotation

Crop rotation is a crucial practice in the field of botany that plays a vital role in maintaining the health and productivity of agricultural systems. It involves systematically changing the type of crops grown in a particular area over time. This technique is based on the principle that different plants have different nutrient requirements and are susceptible to different pests and diseases. By alternating crops, farmers can minimize the buildup of pests and pathogens in the soil, enhance soil fertility, and promote sustainable agriculture.

One of the key benefits of crop rotation is its ability to control pests and diseases. Certain pests and pathogens have a specific host range, meaning they can only survive and reproduce on certain plant species. By rotating crops, farmers disrupt the life cycles of these pests and pathogens, making it difficult for them to establish and spread. This reduces the need for chemical pesticides and helps maintain the overall health of the ecosystem.

In addition to pest and disease control, crop rotation also improves soil fertility. Different crops have different nutrient requirements, and some plants have the ability to fix atmospheric nitrogen, enriching the soil. By diversifying the crops grown in a field, farmers can replenish essential nutrients and prevent the depletion of specific elements. This promotes healthier plant growth and higher yields in the long run.

Furthermore, crop rotation can help manage weeds effectively. Some crops naturally suppress weed growth by shading or competing for resources. By including these crops in the rotation, farmers can reduce weed pressure and minimize the need for herbicides, thus reducing environmental impact.

When implementing crop rotation, it is essential to plan and design a rotation scheme carefully. Factors such as crop compatibility, nutrient requirements, and field conditions should be taken into consideration. By studying the specific needs and characteristics of different crops, students can gain a deeper understanding of the intricate relationships between plants and their environment.

In conclusion, crop rotation is a valuable technique in botany that contributes to sustainable agriculture, pest and disease control, soil fertility, and weed management. By exploring this practice, students can develop a comprehensive understanding of how crop diversity can enhance the health and productivity of agricultural systems.

Crop rotation is a vital practice in the field of botany that plays a crucial role in maintaining the health and productivity of plants. It involves the systematic planting of different crops in a specific order on a piece of land over a period of time. This technique is employed to prevent the buildup of pests, diseases, and nutrient deficiencies that can occur when the same crop is continuously grown in the same area.

The concept of crop rotation is based on the understanding that different plants have varying nutrient requirements and are susceptible to different pests and diseases. By rotating crops, farmers can disrupt the life cycles of pests and pathogens, reducing their populations and preventing the spread of diseases. Additionally, different plants have the ability to extract and absorb different nutrients from the soil. By rotating crops, the nutrient balance in the soil is maintained, ensuring healthy plant growth.

There are several benefits associated with crop rotation. Firstly, it can minimize the need for chemical pesticides and fertilizers as pests and diseases are naturally controlled through the rotation process. This promotes sustainable farming practices and reduces environmental pollution. Secondly, crop rotation enhances soil fertility and structure. Certain crops, such as legumes, have the ability to fix atmospheric nitrogen, enriching the soil with this essential nutrient. Thirdly, it can improve crop yields by reducing the incidence of crop-specific diseases and nutrient deficiencies.

Implementing a crop rotation plan requires careful planning and consideration. Farmers need to select a sequence of crops that are compatible with each other in terms of nutrient requirements and resistance to pests and diseases. It is important to avoid planting crops from the same family consecutively, as they tend to share similar pests and diseases. Instead, farmers should opt for a diverse range of crops to maximize the benefits of rotation.

In conclusion, crop rotation is a fundamental practice in the field of botany that contributes to the overall health and productivity of plants. By strategically rotating crops, farmers can prevent the buildup of pests and diseases, maintain soil fertility, and improve crop yields. It is an essential tool for sustainable farming and plays a significant role in ensuring food security for the future.

Sanitation Measures

In the world of plant pathology, where scientists study the diseases that affect plants, one of the most crucial aspects is implementing effective sanitation measures. These measures play a vital role in preventing the spread of diseases among plants, ensuring their health, and maintaining the overall well-being of our botanical world. As budding botany enthusiasts, it is essential for students to understand the significance of sanitation measures and their role in preserving plant life.

Sanitation measures primarily involve the removal and destruction of infected plant material and the sterilization of tools and equipment used in plant care. These practices help eliminate disease-causing pathogens, such as bacteria, fungi, and viruses, which can harm plants and hinder their growth.

One of the fundamental aspects of sanitation is the removal of infected plant parts. By promptly pruning or removing infected leaves, stems, or fruits, we prevent the disease from spreading to healthy parts of the plant or neighboring plants. It is crucial to properly dispose of the infected material, either by burning it or sealing it in plastic bags before throwing it away. This prevents the pathogens from re-entering the environment and infecting other plants.

Another vital sanitation measure is the sterilization of tools and equipment. Any tools used in gardening or plant care, such as pruning shears, scissors, or containers, should be regularly cleaned and disinfected. This can be done by dipping the tools in a solution of bleach or a disinfectant recommended by experts. Sterilizing tools ensures that pathogens are not unintentionally transferred from one plant to another.

In addition to removing infected plant material and sterilizing tools, maintaining a clean environment around plants is equally important. Regularly cleaning the area around plant beds, removing fallen leaves or debris, and keeping weeds under control helps create a healthy environment for plants to thrive. Weeds often act as reservoirs for plant diseases and can easily spread them to nearby plants.

By implementing these sanitation measures, we can effectively manage and prevent the spread of diseases among plants. As students with a passion for botany, it is crucial to understand the importance of these measures in preserving the health and vitality of our beloved plant kingdom. So, let us embrace these practices and become disease detectives, unraveling the secrets of plant pathology, and ensuring the well-being of our botanical friends.

In the world of botany, where the study of plants and their diseases takes center stage, it is crucial to understand the importance of sanitation measures. Just like humans, plants can also fall prey to various diseases caused by pathogens such as bacteria, fungi, and viruses. These diseases can have devastating effects on crops, gardens, and the overall ecosystem. Therefore, as budding disease detectives in the field of botany, it is essential for students to be well-versed in sanitation measures to prevent and control plant diseases.

Sanitation measures refer to a set of practices aimed at maintaining cleanliness and preventing the spread of pathogens. By implementing these measures, students can minimize the risk of disease transmission and ensure the health and vitality of plants. Let's delve into some key sanitation measures that every botany student should be aware of.

Firstly, practicing good hygiene is paramount. This includes washing hands thoroughly before and after handling plants, as well as sterilizing tools and equipment used in plant care. Disinfecting pruning shears, shovels, and other gardening tools can prevent the transfer of pathogens from one plant to another.

Additionally, maintaining a clean growing environment is essential. Regularly removing fallen leaves, dead plant material, and other debris from the garden or greenhouse can eliminate potential breeding grounds for pathogens. Proper disposal of infected plants is also crucial to prevent the spread of diseases.

Furthermore, crop rotation is a valuable technique to reduce the risk of disease outbreaks. By rotating crops, students can disrupt the life cycle of pathogens that may have built up in the soil. This practice helps to break the cycle of infection and promote healthier plant growth.

Another important aspect of sanitation measures is the careful management of irrigation and watering systems. Overwatering can create a damp environment that fosters the growth of fungi and bacteria. Students should aim to water plants at the base, avoiding wetting the foliage whenever possible.

Lastly, maintaining a healthy balance of nutrients in the soil is vital for plant disease prevention. Providing plants with proper nutrition helps enhance their natural resistance to diseases. Students can achieve this by regularly testing the soil and amending it with organic matter or fertilizers as needed.

By incorporating these sanitation measures into their botany practices, students can become proficient disease detectives, unraveling the secrets of plant pathology. Understanding the significance of sanitation in plant health will not only benefit their studies but also contribute to the larger field of botany and the preservation of our natural ecosystems.

Proper Planting Techniques

When it comes to cultivating healthy plants, proper planting techniques are crucial. Whether you are a student studying botany or simply have a green thumb, understanding how to plant your favorite flowers, vegetables, or trees correctly is essential for their growth and overall well-being. In this subchapter, we will explore some key techniques that will help you become a successful plant cultivator.

First and foremost, it is essential to select the right location for your plants. Different plant species have varying requirements for sunlight, soil type, and moisture levels. Before planting, research the specific needs of your chosen plants to ensure that you place them in an environment where they can thrive. This knowledge will help you create the ideal conditions for their growth and minimize the risk of disease or pest infestation.

Next, preparing the soil properly is crucial. This involves removing any weeds, rocks, or debris and improving the soil's structure and fertility. Adding organic matter, such as compost or well-rotted manure, will enrich the soil and provide vital nutrients for your plants. It is also important to loosen the soil to allow for proper root development and oxygen circulation.

When it comes to planting, it is essential to handle the plants with care. Gently remove them from their containers, being mindful not to damage the roots. If planting seeds, follow the instructions on the seed packet regarding depth and spacing. For transplants, dig a hole slightly larger than the rootball and place the plant in the hole, ensuring it is at the same depth as it was in its original container.

After planting, proper watering is crucial to help the plants establish themselves. Water deeply and thoroughly, ensuring that the root zone receives sufficient moisture. Be mindful not to overwater, as this can lead to root rot and other diseases. It is better to water less frequently but more deeply, allowing the plants to develop a strong root system.

Lastly, it is important to monitor your plants regularly for any signs of disease or pests. Early detection is key to preventing further damage. Learn to identify common plant diseases and pests, and take appropriate measures to control them if necessary. Regularly inspecting your plants and maintaining good hygiene in your garden will go a long way in preventing the spread of diseases.

By following these proper planting techniques, you are setting the foundation for healthy and thriving plants. Remember to always research and understand the specific requirements of your chosen plant species to provide them with the best care possible. Happy gardening!

In the vast world of botany, understanding the importance of proper planting techniques is crucial for any student aspiring to unravel the secrets of plant pathology. Whether you are a beginner or an experienced plant enthusiast, knowing how to plant your greens correctly can make a significant difference in their growth, health, and overall success.

1. Choosing the Right Location: Before digging into the actual planting process, it is essential to select the right location for your plants. Consider factors such as sunlight exposure, soil conditions, and accessibility for watering and

maintenance. Different plant species have specific requirements, so make sure to research and select a spot that meets their needs.

2.   Preparing   the   Soil: Preparing the soil is a fundamental step that ensures your plants receive the necessary nutrients for healthy growth. Remove any weeds, rocks, or debris from the planting area. Loosen the soil using a garden fork or tiller to promote better root penetration and drainage. Adding organic matter, such as compost or well-rotted manure, can improve soil fertility and structure.

3.   Digging   the   Hole: Once the soil is ready, it's time to dig the planting hole. The size and depth of the hole depend on the plant's root system. Generally, the hole should be wider and deeper than the root ball. Gently place the plant in the hole, making sure it sits at the same level it was previously growing.

4.   Backfilling   and   Watering: Carefully backfill the hole with soil, ensuring there are no air pockets around the roots. Lightly tamp down the soil to stabilize the plant. Afterward, water the newly planted greenery thoroughly to help settle the soil and provide hydration. Remember to water regularly, especially during dry periods, to keep the plants healthy.

5.   Mulching   and   Maintenance: Applying a layer of mulch around your plants can help retain moisture, control weeds, and regulate soil temperature. Opt for organic mulches like wood chips or straw, which gradually decompose and enrich the soil. Additionally, regular maintenance practices like

removing dead leaves, providing support for taller plants, and protecting them from pests and diseases are essential for their well-being.

By mastering these proper planting techniques, you will set the stage for successful plant growth and development. Remember to observe your plants closely, as they can provide valuable insights into the fascinating world of plant pathology. Enjoy the journey of unraveling the secrets of plant diseases and how to prevent and combat them. Happy gardening, future disease detectives!

Biological Control Methods

In the fascinating world of plant pathology, disease management is crucial to maintaining healthy plants and crops. One highly effective approach to combating plant diseases is through biological control methods. These methods involve the use of living organisms to control or suppress the populations of plant pathogens, reducing their impact on crops and the environment. In this subchapter, we will explore the various biological control methods used by plant pathologists and their significance in the field of botany.

One widely used biological control method is the introduction of beneficial microorganisms, such as bacteria, fungi, and viruses, to combat plant pathogens. These microorganisms can either directly attack the pathogens or stimulate the plant's natural defense mechanisms, enhancing its ability to resist infection. For example, some bacteria produce compounds that inhibit the growth of harmful fungi, while certain fungi can parasitize and kill pathogenic nematodes in the soil.

Another approach involves the use of beneficial insects, mites, or other arthropods to control plant diseases. These organisms can act as predators, feeding on the pests that transmit diseases or directly attacking the pathogens themselves. Ladybugs, for instance, are well-known for their voracious appetite for aphids, which are notorious carriers of plant viruses.

Additionally, scientists have harnessed the power of plant extracts and natural compounds to control plant diseases. Extracts from certain plants, known as botanicals, contain compounds that exhibit antimicrobial properties against plant pathogens. These botanicals can be used as sprays or incorporated into the soil to protect plants from diseases.

Understanding the interactions between plants, pathogens, and their environment is critical for successful biological control. Plant pathologists conduct extensive research on the ecology and behavior of plant pathogens to develop effective control strategies. By studying the life cycles and vulnerabilities of these pathogens, scientists can identify weak points that can be exploited using biological control methods.

Biological control methods have gained popularity in recent years due to their environmentally friendly nature. Unlike chemical pesticides, which can have detrimental effects on ecosystems, biological control methods pose minimal risks to non-target organisms and the environment.

In conclusion, biological control methods are essential tools in the field of plant pathology. By utilizing living organisms and natural compounds, plant pathologists can effectively manage plant diseases while minimizing harm to the environment. Understanding the principles behind these methods empowers students in the field of botany to contribute to sustainable agriculture and protect the health of our plants and crops for future generations.

In the ever-changing field of botany, one of the most crucial aspects is ensuring the health and vitality of plants. However, plants often face a formidable adversary in the form of pathogens and diseases. To combat these threats, scientists and plant pathologists have developed various methods, one of which is biological control.

Biological control methods involve the use of natural organisms to suppress or eliminate plant diseases. Unlike chemical pesticides that can have harmful effects on the environment, biological control methods are environmentally friendly and sustainable. They utilize beneficial organisms such as bacteria, fungi, viruses, insects, or other microorganisms to control the spread and impact of plant diseases.

One of the most common biological control methods is the use of beneficial bacteria or fungi. These microorganisms, known as biocontrol agents, can outcompete or directly attack the pathogens, preventing their growth and spread. For example, the bacterium Bacillus subtilis has been widely used to control various fungal diseases in crops like tomatoes and cucumbers. Similarly, Trichoderma species of fungi have shown promising results in combating soil-borne pathogens.

Another biological control method involves the use of viruses that specifically target and infect the pathogens. These viruses, called mycoviruses, can disrupt the reproduction and growth of fungal pathogens. By introducing mycoviruses into infected plants, scientists can effectively reduce the severity of the disease.

Insects and other arthropods can also play a significant role in biological control. Predatory insects like lady beetles or parasitic wasps can feed on and control populations of pests that transmit diseases. For instance, certain parasitic wasps lay their eggs inside caterpillars, effectively killing them and preventing further damage to the plant.

To effectively implement biological control methods, scientists conduct extensive research and experiments to identify the most suitable biocontrol agents for specific plant diseases. They also study the interactions between the beneficial organisms, pathogens, and plants to optimize the control strategies.

By utilizing biological control methods, botanists and plant pathologists aim to reduce the reliance on chemical pesticides and promote sustainable practices in agriculture and horticulture. This subchapter explores the fascinating world of biological control and its potential to safeguard plant health, ensuring a greener and healthier future for our planet.

Beneficial Microorganisms

In the world of botany, there is an intricate web of interactions taking place beneath the surface of the soil. While some microbes may cause diseases in plants, there are also numerous beneficial microorganisms that play a crucial role in plant health and growth. These microscopic helpers, often referred to as plant growth-promoting microorganisms (PGPM), have fascinated scientists and researchers for decades, and their importance cannot be overstated.

One group of beneficial microorganisms is the nitrogen-fixing bacteria. These special bacteria have the incredible ability to convert atmospheric nitrogen, which plants cannot utilize directly, into a form that plants can readily absorb. This process, known as nitrogen fixation, provides plants with a vital source of nitrogen, an essential nutrient for their growth and development. By hosting nitrogen-fixing bacteria in their root systems, plants can access this valuable resource and thrive even in nitrogen-poor soils.

Another group of beneficial microorganisms is the mycorrhizal fungi. These fungi establish a symbiotic relationship with plant roots, forming a vast network of filaments called mycelium. Through this network, mycorrhizal fungi enhance the plant's ability to absorb nutrients, especially phosphorus, from the soil. In return, the plants provide the fungi with carbohydrates produced through photosynthesis. This mutualistic partnership not only improves nutrient uptake but also enhances the plant's resistance to diseases and environmental stresses.

Beneficial microorganisms also contribute to plant health by suppressing diseases. Some microorganisms produce antibiotics or other compounds that inhibit the growth of harmful pathogens. They can also stimulate the plant's immune system, making it more resistant to infections. These biocontrol agents offer a sustainable and eco-friendly alternative to chemical pesticides, minimizing the environmental impact and promoting the overall health of the ecosystem.

Understanding the role of beneficial microorganisms in plant pathology is essential for students of botany. By harnessing the power of these microorganisms, scientists and researchers can develop innovative strategies for sustainable agriculture, crop improvement, and disease control. Exploring the intricate relationships between plants and microorganisms opens up a world of possibilities for improving food security and preserving our fragile ecosystems.

In conclusion, beneficial microorganisms are the unsung heroes of the botanical world. From nitrogen-fixing bacteria to mycorrhizal fungi and biocontrol agents, these microscopic allies contribute to plant health, nutrient uptake, and disease suppression. By unraveling the secrets of these microorganisms, students of botany can unlock the potential for sustainable agriculture and make significant contributions to the field of plant pathology.

In the intricate world of botany, there is a hidden army that often goes unnoticed but plays a crucial role in maintaining the health and well-being of plants. These unsung heroes are known as beneficial microorganisms. In this subchapter, we will unravel the secrets of these microscopic allies and explore how they contribute to the field of plant pathology.

Beneficial microorganisms are living organisms that establish a symbiotic relationship with plants. They can be found in various parts of the plant, from the roots to the leaves, and even within the plant cells themselves. One of the most well-known examples of beneficial microorganisms is mycorrhizal fungi. These fungi form a mutually beneficial partnership with the roots of plants, aiding in nutrient uptake and enhancing the plant's ability to withstand stress.

One of the key benefits of these microorganisms is their ability to enhance plant growth and development. They can break down organic matter and release essential nutrients, such as nitrogen and phosphorus, in forms that plants can readily absorb. Additionally, beneficial microorganisms can produce growth-promoting substances, such as hormones and enzymes, which stimulate plant growth and increase resistance to diseases.

Another vital role of beneficial microorganisms is their ability to suppress plant pathogens. They can outcompete harmful microorganisms for resources, produce antimicrobial compounds, and stimulate the plant's natural defense mechanisms. This helps to prevent the establishment and spread of diseases, ultimately leading to healthier and more productive plants.

Furthermore, beneficial microorganisms contribute to the overall health of the soil. They improve soil structure, increase water-holding capacity, and enhance nutrient cycling. By maintaining a balanced microbial community in the soil, these microorganisms help create a favorable environment for plant growth.

As budding botanists, it is crucial to understand the importance of beneficial microorganisms in plant pathology. By harnessing their potential, we can develop sustainable agricultural practices, reduce the reliance on chemical inputs, and promote the health and vitality of plants.

In conclusion, beneficial microorganisms are the unsung heroes of the botanical world. Their symbiotic relationship with plants contributes to plant growth, disease suppression, and overall soil health. By unraveling the secrets of these microscopic allies, we can unlock new possibilities in the field of plant pathology and pave the way for a greener and more sustainable future in botany.

Natural Predators

In the intricate web of nature, where plants play a vital role in sustaining life, there exists a fascinating and often overlooked group of organisms known as natural predators. These remarkable creatures, ranging from insects to birds, play a crucial role in maintaining the delicate balance within the botanical world. As students delving into the captivating realm of botany, understanding the role of natural predators becomes paramount in unraveling the secrets of plant pathology.

In the intricate dance between predator and prey, natural predators have evolved unique adaptations to effectively hunt and control populations of pests that threaten the health of plants. Take, for instance, ladybugs, often adored for their vibrant colors and delicate beauty. These seemingly innocent insects are voracious predators of aphids, a notorious pest that can wreak havoc on plants. By feeding on aphids, ladybugs keep their populations in check, preventing widespread damage to crops and gardens. Observing the behavior and lifecycle of ladybugs can provide valuable insights into the complex dynamics of predator-prey relationships.

Birds also play a significant role in the natural predator community. Many species have developed specialized beaks and feeding techniques to target specific pests. For instance, the woodpecker, with its strong beak, feeds on insects that bore into trees, preventing them from causing extensive damage. Additionally, certain bird species, such as the bluebird, are known to consume large quantities of caterpillars, beetles, and other plant-eating insects. By controlling these pests, birds help maintain the overall health and productivity of plant ecosystems.

Understanding the intricacies of natural predators is not only fascinating but also holds great practical value. As future botanists and scientists, students can harness the knowledge gained from studying natural predators to develop sustainable and environmentally friendly pest control methods. By encouraging the presence of natural predators in agricultural practices, we can reduce our reliance on harmful pesticides, safeguarding both the health of plants and the well-being of our planet.

In conclusion, the subchapter on natural predators opens a window into the captivating world of plant pathology. Exploring the vital role of insects and birds as natural predators not only enriches our understanding of the natural world but also holds immense potential for sustainable pest management practices. As students in the field of botany, embracing the power of natural predators empowers us to protect and preserve the beauty and productivity of our botanical ecosystems.

In the world of plants, just like in the animal kingdom, there are predators lurking in the shadows. These natural predators are not the fierce lions or cunning wolves we often think of, but rather tiny organisms that can cause great harm to plants. In this subchapter, we will explore the fascinating world of natural predators in botany and how they play a crucial role in plant pathology.

One of the most common natural predators in the plant kingdom is fungi. These microscopic organisms are responsible for various plant diseases and can devastate entire crops if left unchecked. Fungi thrive in damp and humid environments, making them a formidable enemy for plants, especially during rainy seasons. They attack plants by invading their tissues, disrupting their normal functions, and eventually causing wilting, rotting, or stunted growth.

Another group of natural predators are bacteria. These tiny single-celled organisms can infect plants through wounds or natural openings, such as stomata. Once inside the plant, bacteria multiply rapidly, leading to the development of diseases like bacterial leaf spots or blights. These diseases can weaken plants, reduce their productivity, and even cause death in severe cases.

Viruses, although not living organisms, are also considered natural predators in the world of botany. Viruses are extremely small and can only replicate inside the cells of a host plant. They are spread through vectors like insects or contaminated tools and can cause a wide range of symptoms, including leaf discoloration, stunted growth, or even complete crop failure. Plant viruses are a major concern for farmers and gardeners worldwide.

While these natural predators may sound like a nightmare for plants, it is important to remember that they are part of a delicate balance in nature. In fact, some predators can be beneficial for plants. For example, certain fungi are used as biocontrol agents to combat harmful plant pathogens. These beneficial fungi colonize plant roots, forming a protective barrier against pathogenic fungi and bacteria.

Understanding the role of natural predators in plant pathology is crucial for botany students. By learning about these organisms and their interactions with plants, students can develop effective strategies to prevent and manage plant diseases. Whether it is through proper cultural practices, the use of resistant plant varieties, or the application of biocontrol agents, students can become disease detectives, unraveling the secrets of plant pathology and safeguarding the health of our green world.

Parasitic Plants

In the vast world of plants, there exists a group of organisms that have evolved a rather unique and cunning way of survival - parasitic plants. These plants, as the name suggests, depend on other plants for their nutrition and growth. They are like plant vampires, stealing vital resources from their hosts to sustain themselves.

Parasitic plants have developed specialized structures called haustoria that enable them to penetrate the tissues of their host plants. Through these haustoria, they establish a connection with the host's vascular system, drawing water, nutrients, and even sugars directly from their hosts. This parasitic lifestyle allows them to bypass the energy-intensive process of photosynthesis, making them highly efficient in their nutrient acquisition.

One well-known example of a parasitic plant is the dodder (Cuscuta species). This plant has thin, twining stems that wrap around its host, forming an intimate connection. Once attached, the dodder sends its haustoria into the host's tissues, tapping into its nutrient-rich sap. The dodder can be quite destructive, causing stunted growth and even death in its victim.

Parasitic plants come in various forms and can target a wide range of host plants. Some species, like mistletoe, live on the branches of trees and shrubs, deriving their nutrients from their hosts. Others, such as the Rafflesia flower, are underground parasites, relying on the roots of nearby plants for sustenance.

While parasitic plants may seem like villains in the plant kingdom, they also play important ecological roles. They can control the growth of certain host plants, preventing them from becoming overly dominant. Additionally, some parasitic plants have been used in traditional medicine for their unique chemical compounds, which may have potential therapeutic applications.

Studying parasitic plants is not only fascinating but also crucial for understanding plant-pathogen interactions and the complex dynamics within ecosystems. Botany students who delve into the world of parasitic plants will gain valuable insights into the strategies these organisms employ to survive and thrive.

In conclusion, parasitic plants are captivating organisms that have evolved specialized mechanisms to survive by siphoning off nutrients from other plants. This subchapter on parasitic plants will explore their unique adaptations, the impact they have on their hosts and ecosystems, and the potential benefits they offer in various fields. By unraveling the secrets of these plant parasites, students will develop a deeper understanding of the intricate world of botany and the fascinating interactions that shape our natural environment.

In the vast world of plant life, there exists a fascinating group of organisms known as parasitic plants. These unique plants have evolved to rely on other plants, known as hosts, for their survival. They have developed remarkable adaptations that allow them to tap into the resources of their hosts, often causing harm in the process. Today, we will delve into the intriguing world of parasitic plants, exploring their characteristics, interactions, and impact on the botanical realm.

Parasitic plants come in various forms, but they all share a common strategy – deriving nutrients and water from their hosts. One well-known example is the dodder, a vine-like parasitic plant that wraps itself around its host and sends out specialized structures called haustoria to penetrate and siphon nutrients from the host's vascular system. Another intriguing case is the mistletoe, which attaches itself to tree branches and taps into the host's water and mineral supply.

These parasitic plants have developed an array of adaptations to survive in their unique lifestyle. For instance, some species have lost their ability to perform photosynthesis, as they obtain their energy directly from their hosts. Others have evolved specialized structures for attachment, such as sucker-like discs or modified roots. Some parasitic plants even mimic the appearance of their hosts' leaves to blend in seamlessly.

The interactions between parasitic plants and their hosts are complex and can have significant consequences. While some hosts can tolerate the presence of parasites, others suffer from stunted growth, reduced vigor, or even death. Parasitic plants can also act as vectors for diseases, further compromising the health of their hosts. Understanding these interactions is crucial for plant pathologists, who study the impact of parasitic plants on agricultural crops and natural ecosystems.

Despite their potentially destructive nature, parasitic plants have intrigued scientists and botanists for centuries. Their unique adaptations and interactions offer valuable insights into the complex web of plant life. By studying these fascinating organisms, students of botany can gain a deeper understanding of the intricate relationships that exist within the plant kingdom.

In conclusion, parasitic plants are a captivating group of organisms that have evolved to rely on other plants for their survival. Their adaptations, interactions, and impacts on the botanical realm make them an intriguing subject for students of botany. By unraveling the secrets of parasitic plants, we can gain a richer understanding of the delicate balance that exists in nature and the complexity of plant pathology.

Chemical Control Measures

In the world of plant pathology, the study of plant diseases, one of the most important aspects is finding effective control measures to combat these diseases. Chemical control measures have proven to be a valuable tool in managing plant diseases and preserving the health and productivity of plants. In this subchapter, we will delve into the realm of chemical control measures and explore how they can help in the field of botany.

Chemical control measures involve the use of various chemicals, such as fungicides, bactericides, and insecticides, to prevent or manage plant diseases. These chemicals work by targeting the pathogens or pests that cause diseases, inhibiting their growth, or killing them outright.

Fungicides are chemicals specifically designed to combat fungal diseases. They are applied to plants as sprays or dusts to prevent fungal spores from germinating or to kill existing fungal infections. Fungicides can be particularly effective in preventing diseases like powdery mildew, rust, and black spot, which commonly afflict plants.

Bactericides, on the other hand, are used to control bacterial diseases. These chemicals work by killing or inhibiting the growth of bacteria that cause diseases such as bacterial blight and fire blight. By using bactericides, botanists can protect plants from devastating bacterial infections.

Insecticides are chemicals designed to control insect pests that can damage or destroy plants. These pests, such as aphids, caterpillars, and beetles, can cause significant harm to crops and gardens. Insecticides can be either contact insecticides, which kill insects upon contact, or systemic insecticides, which are absorbed by the plants and kill insects when they feed on the treated plants.

However, it is important to note that while chemical control measures can be effective, they should be used judiciously and responsibly. Overuse or misuse of chemicals can lead to environmental pollution, harm beneficial insects, and even result in the development of pesticide resistance in pests.

In conclusion, chemical control measures are an important tool in the field of plant pathology. They provide an effective means of managing and preventing plant diseases, aiding in the preservation of plant health and productivity. By understanding the different types of chemicals and their applications, botany students can contribute to the sustainable and responsible use of chemical control measures in the field of plant pathology.

When it comes to protecting plants from diseases, chemical control measures play a crucial role. In this subchapter, we will explore the various methods and strategies used in the field of plant pathology to combat plant diseases through the use of chemicals.

Chemical control measures involve the application of certain substances to either prevent or manage plant diseases. These substances, known as pesticides, can be classified into three main categories: herbicides, fungicides, and insecticides. Each type of pesticide targets specific plant pathogens, such as weeds, fungi, or insects, respectively.

Herbicides are used to control unwanted plants, commonly known as weeds, that compete with crops for nutrients, water, and sunlight. By selectively killing or inhibiting the growth of these plants, herbicides help ensure the health and productivity of cultivated plants. It is important to use herbicides responsibly and in accordance with safety guidelines to minimize any potential negative impact on the environment.

Fungicides, on the other hand, are chemicals designed to combat fungal diseases. Fungi can cause various plant diseases, such as powdery mildew, rust, and blight. Fungicides are formulated to either prevent fungal infections or suppress their growth and spread. It is crucial to identify the specific fungal pathogen affecting the plant in order to choose the most effective fungicide and application method.

Insecticides are used to control insects that can damage plants by feeding on their tissues, transmitting diseases, or causing physical damage. These chemicals can be either contact insecticides, which kill insects upon contact, or systemic insecticides, which are absorbed by the plant and provide long-lasting protection. It is important to use insecticides selectively, targeting only the harmful insects, while preserving beneficial insects that contribute to natural pest control.

While chemical control measures can be effective in managing plant diseases, it is essential to remember that they should be used as part of an integrated pest management (IPM) approach. IPM combines various strategies, including cultural practices, biological control, and chemical control, to minimize the reliance on chemical pesticides. This holistic approach ensures sustainable and environmentally friendly plant disease management.

In conclusion, chemical control measures are an important tool in the field of plant pathology. Herbicides, fungicides, and insecticides help protect plants from weeds, fungal diseases, and harmful insects, respectively. However, their use should be part of an integrated pest management approach to ensure the long-term health and productivity of plants. As students of botany, understanding the principles and responsible use of chemical control measures will enable you to contribute to the field of plant pathology and help safeguard our plant resources for future generations.

Fungicides

Fungi are microscopic organisms that can cause devastating diseases in plants, affecting their growth, development, and overall health. To combat these fungal diseases, scientists and farmers have developed a range of powerful tools, one of which is fungicides. In this subchapter, we will delve into the fascinating world of fungicides and their role in protecting plants from harmful fungal infections.

Fungicides are chemical substances specifically designed to control or eliminate fungal infections in plants. They work by inhibiting or killing the fungi responsible for causing diseases. Different types of fungicides target specific stages of the fungi's life cycle, preventing them from reproducing or damaging the plant further.

There are several classes of fungicides, each with its unique mode of action. Contact fungicides form a protective barrier on the plant's surface, preventing fungal spores from germinating or penetrating the plant tissues. Systemic fungicides, on the other hand, are absorbed by the plant and transported to various parts, including leaves, stems, and roots. They provide long-lasting protection by inhibiting fungal growth from within the plant.

Fungicides can be applied in various forms, such as sprays, dusts, or granules. Farmers and gardeners carefully follow instructions to ensure they apply the correct dosage at the right time. Timing is crucial when using fungicides, as applying them too late may not provide adequate protection, while applying them too early may result in unnecessary chemical use.

It is important to note that while fungicides are effective in combating fungal diseases, they should be used judiciously and as part of an integrated disease management approach. Integrated disease management involves a combination of preventive measures, such as planting disease-resistant varieties, practicing crop rotation, and ensuring proper sanitation in the field or garden.

Students interested in botany and plant pathology can explore the world of fungicides further by studying their environmental impact, potential resistance development in fungi, and ongoing research to develop more sustainable and eco-friendly alternatives. Understanding the proper use and limitations of fungicides will empower future botanists and plant pathologists to develop innovative and sustainable solutions for protecting plants from fungal diseases, ensuring a healthy and productive future for our crops and ecosystems.

In the world of botany, plants face numerous threats, one of which is the presence of harmful fungi. These microscopic organisms can wreak havoc on crops, leading to devastating consequences for farmers and food production. To combat these fungal infections, scientists and farmers have turned to a powerful tool known as fungicides.

Fungicides are chemical substances specifically designed to control or prevent the growth of fungi. These compounds come in various forms, including sprays, dusts, and granules, and are applied directly to plants or their surrounding soil. They work by interfering with the metabolic processes of fungi, inhibiting their growth and reproduction.

One common type of fungicide is the contact fungicide. As the name suggests, contact fungicides act upon direct contact with the fungal pathogen. They form a protective barrier on the plant's surface, preventing the spores from germinating and penetrating the plant's tissues. This type of fungicide is often used as a preventative measure before any signs of infection appear.

Another type of fungicide is the systemic fungicide. Unlike contact fungicides, systemic fungicides are absorbed by the plants and transported throughout their tissues, including the leaves, stems, and roots. As a result, they offer long-lasting protection against fungal infections. Systemic fungicides are particularly useful when dealing with systemic fungal diseases that spread within the plant's vascular system.

It is important to note that while fungicides are effective in controlling fungal infections, they should be used judiciously and as part of an integrated pest management (IPM) strategy. Overuse or misuse of fungicides can lead to the development of resistance in fungi, rendering the chemicals ineffective. Additionally, some fungicides may have adverse effects on non-target organisms, including beneficial insects and microorganisms that contribute to ecosystem health.

To ensure the responsible use of fungicides, it is crucial for students studying botany to understand the principles of plant pathology and the importance of integrated pest management. By incorporating cultural practices, such as crop rotation, sanitation, and proper plant nutrition, along with the targeted application of fungicides, we can effectively manage fungal diseases while minimizing the environmental impact.

In conclusion, fungicides play a vital role in protecting plants from harmful fungal infections. With the knowledge of different types of fungicides and their proper use, students can contribute to sustainable agriculture and help ensure a reliable food supply for future generations. By embracing the principles of plant pathology and integrated pest management, we can become disease detectives, unraveling the secrets of plant pathology and safeguarding the health of our plants.

Bactericides

In the world of plant pathology, bactericides play a crucial role in combating harmful bacteria and protecting our precious plant life. Bacteria are microscopic organisms that can cause devastating diseases in plants, leading to reduced crop yields and economic losses. As budding botanists and students interested in the field of plant pathology, it is important to understand the significance of bactericides and how they contribute to the overall health and well-being of plants.

Bactericides are substances or compounds specifically designed to control or eliminate bacterial infections in plants. They work by targeting the bacteria, disrupting their cellular processes, and ultimately killing or inhibiting their growth. These substances can be classified into two main categories: preventive and curative bactericides.

Preventive bactericides are applied to plants before any signs of bacterial infection are detected. They create a protective barrier on the plant's surface, preventing bacteria from entering and causing damage. Some preventive bactericides are formulated as sprays or coatings that adhere to the plant's leaves, while others are incorporated into the soil to protect the roots. By implementing preventive bactericides, botanists can effectively reduce the risk of bacterial infections and maintain healthy plant populations.

Curative bactericides, on the other hand, are used when plants are already infected with bacteria. They are applied to halt the progression of the disease and limit further damage. Curative bactericides often contain active ingredients that directly target the bacteria, disrupting their growth and preventing them from spreading throughout the plant. These bactericides are typically sprayed onto the infected areas or injected into the plant's vascular system to ensure maximum effectiveness.

It is important to note that while bactericides are powerful tools in the fight against bacterial infections, they should be used judiciously and as part of an integrated pest management approach. Overuse or misuse of bactericides can lead to the development of resistant bacteria strains, making them less effective in the long run. It is crucial for botanists and plant pathologists to employ a combination of cultural practices, genetic resistance, and other pest management strategies alongside bactericides to ensure the sustainable management of bacterial diseases.

In conclusion, bactericides are vital in the field of plant pathology, helping to protect plants from harmful bacterial infections. As students interested in botany and plant pathology, understanding the role of bactericides is essential in our pursuit of unraveling the secrets of plant diseases. By utilizing bactericides wisely and in combination with other management strategies, we can contribute to the sustainable health and prosperity of our plant ecosystems.

Bacteria are microscopic organisms that can cause various diseases in plants, affecting their growth and overall health. In order to protect plants from these harmful bacteria, scientists have developed a range of bactericides. Bactericides are substances or compounds that are specifically designed to inhibit the growth and reproduction of bacteria.

One of the most commonly used bactericides in plant pathology is copper-based compounds. Copper has been found to have antimicrobial properties, making it an effective tool in combating bacterial infections in plants. Copper-based bactericides work by disrupting the cell walls of bacteria, leading to their death. These bactericides are often applied as sprays or dusts on plant surfaces to prevent or control the spread of bacterial diseases.

Another type of bactericide used in plant pathology is antibiotics. Antibiotics are substances derived from living organisms or synthesized in laboratories that can kill or inhibit the growth of bacteria. In agriculture, antibiotics are used to control bacterial diseases in plants. However, it is important to note that the use of antibiotics in agriculture should be carefully regulated to prevent the development of antibiotic-resistant bacteria, which can pose a threat to human health.

Besides copper-based compounds and antibiotics, there are also other bactericides that can be used to combat bacterial diseases in plants. These include biological control agents, such as certain beneficial bacteria and fungi that naturally suppress the growth of harmful bacteria. Biological control agents can be applied to plants to prevent or reduce bacterial infections.

It is important for students studying botany to understand the role of bactericides in plant pathology. By learning about bactericides, students can gain insights into the various strategies used to protect plants from bacterial diseases. Understanding how bactericides work can also help students in their future careers as botanists or plant pathologists, as they may need to develop and implement effective disease management strategies.

In conclusion, bactericides play a vital role in protecting plants from bacterial diseases. Copper-based compounds, antibiotics, and biological control agents are some of the bactericides commonly used in plant pathology. By using these bactericides, scientists and farmers can effectively control bacterial infections and ensure the health and productivity of plants.

Virucides

When it comes to studying plant pathology, it is essential to understand the role of virucides in combating plant viruses. Viruses are microscopic pathogens that infect plants and cause diseases, often resulting in significant damage to crops and vegetation. As students interested in botany, it is crucial to familiarize yourselves with the concept of virucides and their significance in plant disease management.

Virucides are chemical substances specifically designed to kill or inactivate viruses. These powerful agents are used to control and prevent the spread of viral infections in plants. They work by targeting the structure and replication process of viruses, disrupting their ability to infect and multiply within the plant.

One of the most commonly used virucides is bleach. This household chemical is highly effective in killing viruses on surfaces, including gardening tools, pots, and other equipment. However, it is essential to dilute bleach properly and use it in appropriate concentrations to avoid damaging plants. Other virucides include specialized chemical compounds that specifically target plant viruses, offering a more precise and efficient method of virus control.

Apart from chemical virucides, physical methods can also be employed to manage plant viruses. Heat treatments, such as hot water treatment or steam sterilization, can effectively eliminate viruses from plant material, such as seeds or cuttings. This method is commonly used in commercial nurseries and seed banks to ensure disease-free plant propagation.

In recent years, advancements in biotechnology have also resulted in the development of genetically modified plants with increased resistance to specific viruses. These genetically engineered plants produce proteins that interfere with the replication process of the virus, effectively limiting its spread and damage to the plant.

However, it is important to note that the use of virucides should be accompanied by proper cultural practices and integrated pest management strategies. This holistic approach ensures the overall health and well-being of plants, as well as minimizing the reliance on chemical interventions.

As budding botanists, understanding the role of virucides in plant pathology equips us with knowledge to effectively combat plant viruses and preserve the health of our green world. By staying informed about the latest developments in virucide research and implementing responsible plant care practices, we can contribute to the sustainable management of plant diseases and protect our botanical treasures for future generations.

In the vast world of plant pathology, the study of plant diseases, one of the most crucial areas of research is understanding and combating viruses that affect plants. Viruses can wreak havoc on crops, leading to devastating losses in agriculture and threatening food security. It is essential for students interested in botany to grasp the concept of virucides and their role in protecting plants from viral infections.

Virucides, also known as antiviral agents, are substances or treatments that are specifically designed to control or eliminate viruses. These compounds work by targeting the structure or replication process of the virus, effectively inhibiting its ability to infect and spread within plants. Virucides are an integral component of disease management strategies and can significantly reduce the impact of viral diseases on crops.

There are various types of virucides, each with its unique mode of action. Some virucides disrupt the viral envelope, which is the protective outer layer of the virus. By destabilizing this layer, the virucides prevent the virus from entering plant cells and initiating infection. Other virucides interfere with the replication process of the virus, hindering its ability to reproduce and spread throughout the plant.

When it comes to using virucides, it is crucial to follow proper protocols and guidelines to ensure their effectiveness. This includes applying the virucides at the right time, using the correct dosage, and employing proper application techniques. It is also important to consider factors such as the specific virus being targeted, the type of crop, and the environmental conditions to determine the most suitable virucide to use.

Furthermore, it is essential to note that virucides should be used as part of an integrated disease management approach, which includes other practices such as crop rotation, sanitation, and the use of disease-resistant plant varieties. By combining these strategies, farmers and scientists can effectively control viral diseases and protect crops from devastating losses.

For students interested in botany, understanding the role of virucides in plant pathology is crucial. It provides insights into how scientists are actively working to combat viral diseases and protect global food supplies. By studying virucides and their mechanisms of action, students can contribute to the development of innovative solutions for managing viral diseases and ensuring the health and productivity of plants.

Integrated Disease Management Strategies

In the world of botany, disease management plays a crucial role in maintaining the health and productivity of plants. Integrated Disease Management (IDM) strategies have emerged as a comprehensive approach to combating plant diseases, taking into account the complexity of interactions between pathogens, plants, and the environment. This subchapter will explore the various components of IDM strategies and how they can be applied to protect plants and ensure sustainable agriculture.

One key aspect of IDM is the implementation of cultural practices that create unfavorable conditions for disease development. Students will learn about practices such as crop rotation, which involves alternating the cultivation of different plant species in a particular area. This helps break the disease cycle by depriving pathogens of their preferred host plants, thus reducing their populations. Another cultural practice is sanitation, which involves the removal and destruction of diseased plant material to prevent the spread of pathogens.

Biological control is another important component of IDM. Students will discover how beneficial organisms, such as certain bacteria, fungi, and insects, can be employed to suppress plant diseases. They will learn about the concept of antagonism, where these beneficial organisms compete with pathogens for resources, limiting their growth and spread. This natural approach to disease management is not only environmentally friendly but also sustainable in the long term.

Chemical control, while not the sole focus of IDM, can also be a valuable tool when used judiciously. Students will gain an understanding of the principles of pesticide use, including the importance of correctly identifying the pest or pathogen and choosing the appropriate product. They will also learn about the significance of following label instructions and adhering to safety guidelines to minimize environmental impacts.

Furthermore, students will explore the concept of host plant resistance, which involves breeding plants with inherent resistance to specific diseases. They will discover how researchers employ techniques such as genetic engineering and traditional breeding to develop resistant varieties that can withstand infection and reduce the need for chemical interventions.

By delving into the realm of Integrated Disease Management strategies, students will gain a comprehensive understanding of the multifaceted approaches used to combat plant diseases. They will appreciate the importance of cultural practices, biological control, chemical control, and host plant resistance in ensuring the health and productivity of plants and sustaining our agricultural systems. Armed with this knowledge, they will be well-equipped to become disease detectives, unraveling the secrets of plant pathology and contributing to the future of botany.

In the fascinating world of botany, understanding and managing plant diseases is essential for a successful and sustainable agriculture system. As students in the field of botany, it is crucial to unravel the secrets of plant pathology and learn about integrated disease management strategies that can help combat these challenges. This subchapter aims to introduce you to some of the effective strategies used in integrated disease management.

Integrated disease management (IDM) is a holistic approach that combines various strategies to control and prevent plant diseases. It emphasizes the use of multiple tools and techniques to reduce disease incidence and severity, while also minimizing the negative impact on the environment. IDM strategies often involve cultural, biological, and chemical methods, all working together to create a balanced and resilient plant ecosystem.

One of the key aspects of IDM is cultural practices. These practices involve manipulating the environment to create conditions that are unfavorable for disease development. This can include crop rotation, which helps break disease cycles by planting different crops in a specific sequence. Another cultural practice is proper sanitation, which involves removing infected plant debris and cleaning tools and equipment to prevent disease spread.

Biological control is another important IDM strategy. It involves using beneficial organisms, such as predators, parasites, and pathogens, to suppress disease-causing organisms. These organisms act as natural enemies of the pathogens, helping to reduce their population and limit disease progression. For example, introducing predatory insects that feed on plant pests can help control the spread of diseases transmitted by these pests.

Chemical control methods, such as the use of fungicides, are also part of IDM strategies. However, these methods should be used judiciously and as a last resort, as they can have adverse effects on the environment and human health. It is crucial to follow label instructions and apply chemicals only when necessary and in the recommended dosage.

In conclusion, integrated disease management strategies are vital for effective plant disease control in the field of botany. By combining cultural practices, biological control, and judicious use of chemicals, we can create a sustainable and resilient plant ecosystem. As students, understanding and implementing these strategies will not only contribute to our knowledge of botany but also help ensure the health and well-being of our plants and environment.

Chapter 6: Disease Detection and Surveillance

Importance of Early Detection

In the vast world of botany, understanding the importance of early detection in plant pathology is crucial. As students embarking on a journey to unravel the secrets of plant diseases, you are equipped with the knowledge to become disease detectives, safeguarding the health and productivity of plants. This subchapter delves into the significance of early detection in the field of botany and why it plays a vital role in combating plant diseases.

Early detection refers to the identification of signs and symptoms of diseases at their early stages. By recognizing these indicators, scientists and botanists can take prompt action to prevent the spread of diseases and minimize their impact on plants. Early detection serves as the first line of defense against plant pathogens, ensuring the health and survival of our green friends.

One of the primary reasons early detection is crucial is its potential to save crops and protect food security. Plant diseases can devastate entire fields, resulting in significant economic losses and food shortages. By detecting diseases early on, scientists can implement strategies such as quarantine measures, disease-resistant crop varieties, or targeted treatments to prevent the rapid spread of pathogens. This proactive approach not only safeguards the livelihoods of farmers but also ensures a stable supply of food for our growing population.

Moreover, early detection allows scientists to study the biology and behavior of plant pathogens more comprehensively. By closely monitoring the progression of diseases, researchers can gain valuable insights into the mechanisms employed by pathogens, their life cycles, and environmental factors that influence their growth. This knowledge is essential for developing effective control strategies, including the creation of resistant crop varieties or the formulation of environmentally friendly biocontrol methods.

Early detection also plays a crucial role in conservation efforts. Many plant species are threatened by diseases, leading to biodiversity loss and ecological imbalances. By swiftly identifying diseases in endangered plant populations, conservationists can take immediate action to protect these species from extinction. Early detection allows for targeted interventions, such as implementing protective measures or initiating restoration programs, ensuring the preservation of our planet's botanical diversity.

In conclusion, early detection is of utmost importance in the field of botany. As students and aspiring disease detectives, recognizing the signs and symptoms of plant diseases is vital in safeguarding crop productivity, ensuring food security, protecting biodiversity, and advancing our understanding of plant pathogens. By unraveling the secrets of plant pathology, you have the power to make a significant impact in the world of botany and contribute to the well-being of our planet.

One of the fundamental aspects of plant pathology that every aspiring botanist should understand is the importance of early detection in preventing and managing diseases. Detecting diseases in plants at their earliest stages is crucial for maintaining the health and vitality of our botanical world. In this subchapter, we will dive into the significance of early detection and explore the various strategies and tools that can be utilized to identify and combat plant diseases.

Early detection plays a pivotal role in preventing widespread outbreaks of plant diseases. Just like in human health, prompt identification of diseases in plants allows for timely intervention, minimizing the damage caused and preventing further spread. By detecting diseases early, students of botany can effectively employ appropriate control measures, such as targeted treatments and quarantine protocols, to contain and manage the affected plants or areas.

Moreover, early detection can help botanists understand the underlying causes and mechanisms of plant diseases. By closely observing and monitoring the initial symptoms, students can gain insights into the pathogen's life cycle, modes of transmission, and host range. This knowledge is invaluable in developing effective management strategies, breeding resistant varieties, and implementing preventive measures to protect our cherished plant species.

To achieve early detection, students must be equipped with the necessary tools and techniques. The use of advanced diagnostic methods, such as molecular markers, DNA sequencing, and microscopy, allows for accurate and rapid identification of plant pathogens. Students can also learn how to recognize typical symptoms and signs of diseases, such as wilting, discoloration, lesions, or abnormal growth patterns, during their botanical studies. With these skills, they can become disease detectives who play a vital role in safeguarding the health of our botanical world.

In conclusion, the importance of early detection in plant pathology cannot be overstated. By promptly identifying and addressing diseases in their early stages, students of botany can protect plants from extensive damage, prevent widespread outbreaks, and contribute to the preservation of our botanical diversity. Early detection also provides crucial insights into the nature of plant diseases, guiding the development of effective management strategies. As future botanists and disease detectives, it is essential for students to understand and embrace the significance of early detection in their pursuit of unraveling the secrets of plant pathology.

Methods of Disease Surveillance

In the world of plant pathology, disease surveillance plays a crucial role in identifying, monitoring, and preventing the spread of harmful plant diseases. By understanding the methods of disease surveillance, students studying botany can become disease detectives themselves, unraveling the secrets of plant pathology and safeguarding the health of our green friends.

One of the most common methods of disease surveillance is visual inspections. Students can learn to identify visual symptoms and signs of diseases on plants. Symptoms include wilting, discoloration, leaf spots, and deformities, while signs may include fungal fruiting bodies or insect pests. By regularly inspecting plants, students can detect diseases early on and take necessary actions to prevent their spread.

Another method is the use of diagnostic tests. Students can learn to conduct laboratory tests to identify the pathogens responsible for causing diseases. This involves collecting samples from infected plants, isolating the pathogens, and growing them on culture media. Through techniques such as microscopy, DNA analysis, and serological tests, students can accurately identify the specific pathogens involved and determine the best management strategies.

Surveillance can also be done through the use of remote sensing technologies. Students can explore the use of satellite imagery, drones, and other advanced tools to detect changes in plant health over large areas. By analyzing the data collected, students can identify areas where diseases may be spreading rapidly and take preventive measures accordingly.

Additionally, students can learn about the importance of disease reporting systems. They can understand how to report the occurrence and spread of diseases to their local agricultural extension services or plant health authorities. This information helps in the timely implementation of control measures and prevents further damage to crops and natural ecosystems.

Lastly, students can explore the power of citizen science in disease surveillance. By actively participating in programs like Plant-Pathogen Watch, students can contribute their observations and data to a wider network of scientists and researchers. This collaborative effort enhances disease surveillance capabilities and helps in better understanding the dynamics of plant diseases.

In conclusion, disease surveillance is an essential aspect of plant pathology, and students studying botany can actively participate in this field by utilizing various methods. By honing their skills in visual inspections, diagnostic tests, remote sensing, disease reporting, and citizen science, students can become proficient disease detectives, unraveling the secrets of plant pathology, and contributing to the health and sustainability of our plant ecosystems.

In the captivating world of botany, disease surveillance plays a crucial role in unraveling the secrets of plant pathology. By understanding and implementing various methods, scientists can detect, monitor, and control diseases that affect our beloved plants. This subchapter will delve into the fascinating methods used in disease surveillance, providing students with a comprehensive overview of this essential field.

One of the primary methods employed in disease surveillance is visual inspection. By closely examining plants, scientists can identify symptoms such as wilting, discoloration, lesions, or abnormal growth patterns. This simple yet effective method allows for the early detection of diseases, enabling prompt action to mitigate their spread.

To complement visual inspection, laboratory techniques are also employed. Scientists extract samples from infected plants and analyze them under microscopes to identify specific pathogens. By studying the characteristics of these disease-causing agents, researchers can determine the most appropriate control measures, including the development of resistant plant varieties or targeted treatments.

In recent years, technological advancements have revolutionized disease surveillance in botany. Remote sensing techniques, such as drones equipped with high-resolution cameras, allow scientists to monitor large areas quickly and efficiently. These aerial surveys provide valuable data on plant health, enabling early detection of diseases over vast landscapes.

Furthermore, molecular methods have become indispensable in disease surveillance. Polymerase Chain Reaction (PCR) is a widely used technique that amplifies DNA fragments specific to certain pathogens, enabling their detection even in small amounts. This method provides accurate and rapid results, aiding in the identification and tracking of diseases.

Another innovative approach is the use of data analytics and machine learning algorithms. By collecting and analyzing vast amounts of data, scientists can identify patterns and correlations between environmental factors, plant health, and disease outbreaks. This knowledge helps predict disease occurrences and improves prevention strategies in a proactive manner.

In conclusion, disease surveillance in botany relies on a variety of methods that combine traditional techniques and cutting-edge technologies. Visual inspection, laboratory analysis, remote sensing, molecular methods, and data analytics all contribute to the early detection, monitoring, and control of plant diseases. By studying and implementing these methods, students interested in botany can become disease detectives, playing a vital role in unraveling the secrets of plant pathology and ensuring the health and vitality of our plant life.

Visual Inspections

In the fascinating world of plant pathology, visual inspections play a crucial role in unraveling the secrets of plant diseases. As budding disease detectives, it is essential for students with an interest in botany to master the art of visual inspections. By closely observing plants and their symptoms, you can uncover vital clues that will help you understand and combat plant diseases effectively.

Visual inspections involve carefully examining plants for any abnormalities or signs of distress. These signs can manifest in various ways, such as discoloration, wilting, stunted growth, or unusual spots on leaves or stems. As students in the field of botany, it is important to develop a keen eye for detail and learn to differentiate between healthy and diseased plants.

To conduct a visual inspection, start by selecting a few plants for observation. Look for any visible symptoms and note them down in detail. Pay attention to the color, texture, and shape of leaves, stems, flowers, and fruits. Examine the roots for any signs of rot or discoloration. Engage all your senses during the inspection - observe the appearance, feel the texture, and even smell for any unusual odors.

While conducting visual inspections, it is crucial to keep in mind that plant diseases can be caused by various factors, including bacteria, fungi, viruses, or environmental stressors. Therefore, it is essential to observe not only the affected plants but also their surroundings. Take note of any changes in temperature, humidity, or water availability, as these factors can influence the development and spread of plant diseases.

Visual inspections also involve monitoring plants over time. Record the progression of symptoms, noting any changes or new symptoms that appear. This longitudinal observation will help you determine the severity of the disease and track its spread. Additionally, it will provide valuable insights into the effectiveness of any treatments or management strategies employed.

By mastering the technique of visual inspections, students in the field of botany can become skilled disease detectives. These inspections will enable you to identify and diagnose plant diseases accurately, leading to effective measures for disease prevention and control. So, grab your magnifying glasses and venture into the world of visual inspections to unravel the secrets of plant pathology!

In the realm of botany, visual inspections play a crucial role in unraveling the secrets of plant pathology. As students exploring the fascinating world of plant diseases, it is important to develop the skills of keen observation and careful examination. In this subchapter, we will dive into the realm of visual inspections and discover how they can help us identify and understand plant diseases.

Visual inspections involve closely examining plants for any signs or symptoms of disease. These signs can be seen on various plant parts, including leaves, stems, flowers, and fruits. By observing these signs, we can gather valuable information about the type of pathogen or pest affecting the plant and the stage of the disease.

To begin a visual inspection, it is essential to choose healthy plants as reference points for comparison. By comparing healthy plants to potentially diseased ones, we can easily identify any abnormalities.

Look for changes in color, texture, size, or shape of plant parts. Discoloration, spots, wilting, deformities, or any other unusual characteristics can serve as red flags indicating the presence of a disease.

While conducting visual inspections, it is important to consider the time of day and lighting conditions. Shadows can sometimes obscure certain symptoms or signs, so it is recommended to inspect plants during daylight hours. Take your time and inspect each plant individually, examining both the upper and lower surfaces of leaves, stems, and other plant parts.

It is also crucial to note any patterns or distribution of symptoms. Are the symptoms localized or spread throughout the plant? Are they concentrated in specific areas? Such observations can provide valuable insights into the mode of disease spread and the potential pathogen involved.

Throughout the visual inspection process, it is essential to document your findings. Take clear photographs or make detailed sketches of the observed symptoms and signs. These records will serve as valuable references for future comparisons and discussions with experts in the field of plant pathology.

Visual inspections are an indispensable tool for budding botanists and plant pathologists. By honing your observation skills and carefully examining plants, you can unravel the secrets of plant diseases and contribute to the field of botany. So, grab your magnifying glass and embark on the journey of visual inspections to unlock the mysteries of plant pathology!

Remote Sensing Techniques

In the vast field of botany, the use of remote sensing techniques has revolutionized the way we study plant pathology. Remote sensing involves the collection and analysis of data from a distance, without physically touching the subject. This innovative approach has allowed scientists and researchers to gain a deeper understanding of plant diseases and their impact on the environment. In this subchapter, we will explore the various remote sensing techniques used in plant pathology research.

One of the most commonly used remote sensing techniques is aerial photography. By capturing images from aircraft or satellites, scientists can monitor large areas of vegetation and identify patterns associated with disease outbreaks. Aerial photographs provide valuable information about plant health, such as changes in color or texture, which can indicate the presence of pathogens. This technique allows for the rapid detection and mapping of disease spread, aiding in the development of effective control strategies.

Another powerful remote sensing tool is hyperspectral imaging. This technique involves capturing images at multiple wavelengths, allowing researchers to analyze the spectral signature of plants. Each plant disease has a unique spectral signature, which can be detected using hyperspectral imaging. By comparing healthy and infected plants, scientists can accurately identify and monitor diseases, even before visible symptoms appear. Hyperspectral imaging has proven to be highly effective in identifying pathogens and assessing their impact on plant health.

Furthermore, thermal imaging is a remote sensing technique that measures the heat emitted by plants. Infected plants often exhibit changes in temperature due to physiological responses to pathogens. By using thermal imaging cameras, researchers can detect these temperature variations and identify areas of infection. This technique not only helps in pinpointing disease hotspots but also aids in understanding the progression of infections and their effects on plant physiology.

Lastly, LiDAR (Light Detection and Ranging) technology has found its application in plant pathology research. LiDAR uses laser pulses to measure the distance between the sensor and the target, creating highly accurate 3D models of vegetation. By analyzing these models, researchers can detect changes in plant structure caused by diseases. LiDAR allows for the quantification of disease severity and aids in understanding its impact on plant growth and development.

In conclusion, remote sensing techniques have revolutionized the field of plant pathology by providing valuable insights into the detection, monitoring, and management of plant diseases. Aerial photography, hyperspectral imaging, thermal imaging, and LiDAR are just a few examples of the powerful tools at our disposal. As budding botanists, understanding and harnessing the potential of remote sensing techniques will enable us to unravel the secrets of plant pathology and contribute to the protection and conservation of our precious botanical resources.

In the world of botany, understanding the health and well-being of plants is crucial for their growth and survival. As students exploring the fascinating field of plant pathology, it is essential to unravel the secrets hidden within the plant kingdom. One powerful tool that can help us achieve this is remote sensing techniques.

Remote sensing involves the use of various technologies to gather information about an object or area without direct physical contact. In the context of botany, this technique allows scientists to monitor and study plants from a distance, providing valuable insights into their health, growth patterns, and the presence of pathogens.

One commonly used remote sensing technique is aerial photography. By capturing images of plants from above using drones or aircraft, scientists can observe changes in plant color, density, and structure. These images can then be analyzed to identify patterns indicative of plant diseases or stress. For example, a sudden change in leaf color or a decrease in plant density may suggest the presence of a pathogen.

Another remote sensing technique is hyperspectral imaging. This technology involves capturing and analyzing the reflectance of light across a wide range of wavelengths. Each plant species has a unique spectral signature, which can be used to identify specific diseases or nutrient deficiencies. By measuring the reflectance of light, scientists can detect subtle changes in plant health that may not be visible to the naked eye.

Satellite imagery is yet another valuable remote sensing tool for studying plants. Satellites equipped with sensors can provide a vast amount of data on vegetation indices, such as the Normalized Difference Vegetation Index (NDVI). These indices indicate the overall health and vigor of plants, helping scientists to monitor large-scale changes in vegetation over time. Satellite imagery is particularly useful for detecting widespread plant diseases or environmental stressors that affect entire regions.

Remote sensing techniques offer students of botany a unique and powerful way to explore the secrets of plant pathology. By harnessing the capabilities of aerial photography, hyperspectral imaging, and satellite imagery, we can gain a deeper understanding of plant health, identify diseases, and develop effective management strategies. As we delve further into the world of botany, let us embrace these remote sensing techniques as invaluable tools in our quest to unravel the mysteries of plant pathology.

Molecular Tools for Surveillance

In the exciting world of plant pathology, scientists are constantly on the hunt for new ways to detect and monitor diseases in plants. One of the most powerful tools they use is molecular surveillance. By harnessing the power of molecular biology, plant pathologists can identify and track the presence of harmful pathogens in order to protect our crops and ensure food security.

Molecular surveillance involves the use of various techniques to detect and analyze the DNA or RNA of plant pathogens. This allows scientists to identify specific pathogens quickly and accurately, even before visible symptoms appear in the plants. By doing so, they can take proactive measures to prevent the spread of diseases and minimize crop losses.

One of the most commonly used molecular tools for surveillance is polymerase chain reaction (PCR). PCR allows scientists to amplify a specific DNA sequence from a small sample, making it easier to detect the presence of pathogens. This technique has revolutionized plant pathology by enabling rapid and accurate diagnosis of diseases. Students can think of PCR as a magnifying glass that helps scientists see the invisible world of pathogens.

Another powerful molecular tool is DNA sequencing. By determining the precise order of nucleotides in a pathogen's DNA, scientists can compare it to known sequences and identify the exact species or strain responsible for the disease. This information is invaluable for tracking the origin and spread of pathogens, giving scientists valuable insights into disease dynamics.

To make the most of these molecular tools, scientists often rely on bioinformatics. This interdisciplinary field combines biology, computer science, and statistics to analyze and interpret vast amounts of genetic data. By using specialized software and algorithms, plant pathologists can identify patterns and relationships between different pathogens, helping them develop effective strategies for disease management.

As budding botanists, understanding the role of molecular tools in disease surveillance is crucial. By learning about these cutting-edge techniques, you can contribute to the field of plant pathology and help protect our precious plant resources. With the power of molecular biology, we can unravel the secrets of plant diseases and stay one step ahead in the fight against pathogens.

In the world of plant pathology, surveillance plays a crucial role in detecting and preventing the spread of diseases that can devastate crops and natural ecosystems. Traditional methods of surveillance involve visual inspections and sample collection, but in recent years, molecular tools have revolutionized the field. These powerful tools provide scientists with faster and more accurate methods for identifying pathogens and monitoring their movements.

One of the most widely used molecular tools for surveillance is polymerase chain reaction (PCR). PCR allows scientists to amplify and study specific DNA sequences, enabling the identification of pathogens even in low quantities. By comparing the DNA sequences obtained from samples with known sequences of pathogens, researchers can quickly determine if a particular disease-causing agent is present. PCR has proven to be invaluable in diagnosing plant diseases and monitoring their spread, allowing for timely interventions to prevent further damage.

Another important molecular tool is DNA barcoding. This technique involves sequencing a short, standardized region of DNA from a specimen to identify its species. By comparing the obtained sequence with a reference database, scientists can accurately identify the pathogen responsible for a disease outbreak. DNA barcoding is particularly useful for identifying pathogens that are difficult to distinguish based on their morphology alone, providing a rapid and reliable method for surveillance.

Advancements in next-generation sequencing (NGS) technologies have also greatly enhanced surveillance capabilities. NGS allows scientists to simultaneously sequence millions of DNA fragments, providing a comprehensive view of the microbial community present in a sample. This approach, known as metagenomics, enables the detection of known and unknown pathogens, as well as the identification of potential emerging threats. NGS-based surveillance has the potential to revolutionize plant pathology by providing a deeper understanding of the complex interactions between plants, pathogens, and the environment.

As students interested in botany, understanding the importance of molecular tools for surveillance is crucial. These tools not only enable early detection and accurate identification of plant pathogens, but also inform the development of effective management strategies. By staying informed about the latest advancements in molecular tools, you can contribute to the field of plant pathology and help protect our crops and natural ecosystems from devastating diseases.

Chapter 7: Case Studies in Plant Pathology

Major Plant Diseases and Outbreaks

As students of botany, it is essential to understand the major plant diseases and outbreaks that can have a significant impact on agricultural productivity and plant health. In this subchapter, we will explore some of the most common and destructive plant diseases, their causes, and the measures that can be taken to prevent or manage them.

One of the most notorious plant diseases is the fungal infection called powdery mildew. This disease affects a wide range of plants, including roses, cucumbers, and grapes, leaving a powdery white coating on the leaves and stems. Powdery mildew thrives in humid conditions and can spread rapidly, causing severe damage to crops if left unchecked. To prevent powdery mildew outbreaks, it is crucial to maintain proper ventilation and avoid overwatering plants.

Another significant plant disease is the bacterial infection known as fire blight. This disease primarily affects fruit trees such as apples and pears, causing wilting, blackening of branches, and a scorched appearance. Fire blight spreads through insects, rain, or pruning tools, making it important to sanitize tools and remove infected plant parts promptly. Some resistant plant varieties and regular pruning can also help prevent the spread of fire blight.

A viral disease that poses a threat to many crops is the Tomato Yellow Leaf Curl Virus (TYLCV). This virus affects tomato plants, causing yellowing and curling of leaves, stunted growth, and reduced yields. TYLCV is transmitted by whiteflies and can quickly devastate entire tomato crops. Implementing integrated pest management strategies, such as using reflective mulches and releasing beneficial insects, can help control whitefly populations and reduce the spread of TYLCV.

In addition to these specific diseases, other major plant disease outbreaks have had a significant impact on global agriculture. For example, the Irish Potato Famine in the 19th century was caused by a fungal disease called late blight, which destroyed potato crops, leading to widespread famine and migration. Understanding the history and consequences of such outbreaks emphasizes the importance of plant disease research and management.

By learning about major plant diseases and outbreaks, students of botany can develop a deeper understanding of the challenges faced by farmers and plant pathologists. This knowledge can help in developing strategies to prevent, manage, and mitigate the impact of these diseases, ultimately contributing to sustainable agriculture and global food security.

In the fascinating world of botany, the study of plants, there exists an intricate relationship between plants and diseases. Just as humans and animals can fall sick, plants too can be affected by various diseases caused by harmful microorganisms. These diseases can spread rapidly, leading to outbreaks that can devastate entire crops and landscapes. In this subchapter, we will explore some of the major plant diseases and outbreaks that have had a significant impact on our agricultural systems.

One of the most notorious plant diseases is the Irish potato famine, which occurred in the mid-19th century. Phytophthora infestans, a water mold, caused widespread destruction of potato crops in Ireland, resulting in a devastating famine that claimed the lives of millions of people. This outbreak serves as a stark reminder of the importance of plant disease research and prevention.

Another notable plant disease is the Panama disease, caused by the fungus Fusarium oxysporum. This disease affects banana plants, causing wilting and eventually killing the entire plant. Panama disease has had a significant impact on the global banana industry, as it spreads easily and can wipe out entire plantations.

Citrus canker, caused by the bacterium Xanthomonas citri subsp. citri, is a major concern for citrus growers worldwide. This disease leads to the formation of characteristic corky lesions on the leaves, fruit, and stems of citrus trees, reducing their productivity and quality. Efforts to control and prevent citrus canker outbreaks are crucial for maintaining healthy citrus orchards.

In recent years, the emergence of new plant diseases has raised concerns among botanists and agricultural scientists. One such example is the sudden oak death, caused by the oomycete Phytophthora ramorum. This disease primarily affects oak trees and has spread to various regions worldwide, leading to the death of millions of oaks and impacting forest ecosystems.

Understanding the causes, symptoms, and management strategies for major plant diseases is essential for students interested in botany. As future botanists and plant pathologists, students play a vital role in mitigating the impact of plant diseases on our food security and ecosystem health. By studying these diseases, students can contribute to the development of innovative strategies for disease prevention, early detection, and effective management.

In conclusion, major plant diseases and outbreaks pose significant challenges to the field of botany. By unraveling the secrets of plant pathology, students can become disease detectives, helping to protect our plants, crops, and ecosystems from devastating diseases.

The Irish Potato Famine

The Irish Potato Famine was a devastating event that occurred in Ireland between 1845 and 1852. It was caused by a plant disease known as late blight, which affected the potato crop, upon which the majority of the Irish population heavily relied. This subchapter of "Disease Detectives: Unraveling the Secrets of Plant Pathology for Students" aims to shed light on the causes, effects, and lessons learned from the Irish Potato Famine, catering specifically to students interested in botany.

Late blight, caused by the pathogen Phytophthora infestans, is a fungal-like organism that thrives in cool, wet environments. It infects the leaves and stems of potato plants, turning them brown and causing the tubers to rot. The disease spreads rapidly, leading to the decimation of entire potato crops. With potatoes being a staple food in Ireland at the time, the failure of this crop had severe consequences for the population.

The impact of the Irish Potato Famine was catastrophic. Over a million people died from starvation or related diseases, and many more were forced to emigrate in search of a better life. The social, economic, and political landscape of Ireland was forever changed. The famine also exposed the vulnerability of relying heavily on a single crop for sustenance, highlighting the importance of crop diversity and disease resistance in agriculture.

One of the lessons learned from the Irish Potato Famine is the significance of plant pathology in agricultural practices. Plant pathologists study plant diseases and develop strategies to manage and control them. By understanding the causes and mechanisms of plant diseases, scientists can develop resistant crop varieties and implement disease management practices to prevent similar catastrophes.

Furthermore, the Irish Potato Famine demonstrated the need for sustainable agricultural practices. Monoculture, or the practice of growing a single crop on a large scale, increases the risk of disease outbreaks. Crop rotation, where different crops are grown in succession, helps break the disease cycle and maintains soil health. Integrated pest management, which combines various strategies to control pests and diseases, is another important approach to safeguarding crops.

In conclusion, the Irish Potato Famine serves as a tragic reminder of the devastating consequences of plant diseases and the importance of plant pathology in preventing such disasters. As students interested in botany, it is crucial to understand the significance of crop diversity, disease resistance, and sustainable agricultural practices in ensuring food security and preventing future catastrophes. By studying plant pathology, you can play a vital role in protecting our crops and securing a sustainable future for agriculture.

The Irish Potato Famine is one of the most devastating events in history, with profound consequences for Ireland and its people. This subchapter will delve into the causes, impact, and lessons learned from this tragic period, shedding light on the field of plant pathology and its relevance to students interested in botany.

In the mid-19th century, Ireland heavily relied on potatoes as a staple crop due to their high productivity and nutritional value. However, disaster struck when a devastating plant disease known as late blight, caused by the pathogen Phytophthora infestans, ravaged potato fields across the country. This highly contagious disease quickly spread, infecting and destroying potato plants, leading to severe food shortages and famine.

The impact of the Irish Potato Famine was catastrophic. Millions of people faced starvation and malnutrition, resulting in mass emigration, death, and social upheaval. This event not only highlighted the vulnerability of relying heavily on a single crop but also the importance of understanding plant diseases and their management.

Plant pathology, a branch of botany, seeks to unravel the secrets of plant diseases and find ways to protect crops. By studying the Irish Potato Famine, students can gain a deeper understanding of the importance of plant health and the need for disease detection and management strategies. They will learn about the lifecycle of plant pathogens, their modes of transmission, and the impact they can have on agricultural systems.

Furthermore, the Irish Potato Famine serves as a reminder of the importance of diversifying crop choices and implementing disease management practices. Students interested in botany can explore the various methods used to combat plant diseases, such as breeding resistant crop varieties, implementing cultural practices, and developing chemical and biological controls.

By studying the Irish Potato Famine, students can also develop critical thinking skills as they analyze the actions taken during the crisis and evaluate the long-term impacts on agriculture and society. They can gain an appreciation for the interconnectedness of plant health, food security, and social well-being.

In conclusion, the Irish Potato Famine is a significant event in history that provides valuable lessons for students interested in botany. By understanding the causes and consequences of this devastating event, students can appreciate the importance of plant pathology in safeguarding crop health and explore ways to address future plant diseases and their impact on society.

Dutch Elm Disease

Disease Detectives: Unraveling the Secrets of Plant Pathology for Students

Botany students, welcome to the fascinating world of plant pathology! In this subchapter, we will delve into a notorious disease that has had a devastating impact on Elm trees worldwide - Dutch Elm Disease (DED).

Dutch Elm Disease is caused by a fungus called Ophiostoma novo-ulmi, which is primarily spread by the elm bark beetle. This disease was first identified in the Netherlands in the early 20th century and quickly spread across Europe and North America. It has since become one of the most destructive tree diseases in the world.

So, how does Dutch Elm Disease affect Elm trees? The fungus invades the tree through wounds created by the beetle's feeding activity. Once inside, it multiplies and spreads, blocking the tree's vascular system, which is responsible for transporting water and nutrients. As a result, the tree's leaves wilt, turn yellow, and eventually die. Without prompt action, infected trees can die within a few short years.

Understanding the life cycle of the fungus and the beetle is crucial for preventing the spread of Dutch Elm Disease. Researchers have discovered that the fungus produces spores that are carried by the beetles from infected trees to healthy ones. This means that controlling the beetle population is essential in managing the disease. Arborists and scientists have developed various strategies to combat Dutch Elm Disease, including the use of insecticides to kill the beetles and injecting fungicides or antibiotics into infected trees to slow down the disease progression.

To prevent the spread of Dutch Elm Disease, early detection is key. Students of botany can contribute to disease management by learning to identify the symptoms of DED, such as wilting leaves, brown streaks in the wood, and discoloration of the bark. By reporting potential cases to local authorities or arborists, students can play a crucial role in preventing further spread and saving healthy Elm trees.

In conclusion, Dutch Elm Disease is a devastating fungal disease that has significantly impacted Elm trees worldwide. As students of botany, understanding the disease's causes, symptoms, and management strategies is essential for preserving our natural ecosystems. By being vigilant and proactive in reporting potential cases, you can contribute to the ongoing efforts in combating Dutch Elm Disease and protecting our beloved Elm trees for generations to come.

Dutch Elm Disease is a devastating plant disease that has had a significant impact on elm trees worldwide. This subchapter aims to introduce students to the basics of this disease, its causes, symptoms, and potential prevention methods.

Caused by a fungus called Ophiostoma ulmi, Dutch Elm Disease spreads through the transportation of infected wood or bark beetles. The disease primarily affects elm trees, which are known for their majestic appearance and importance in the ecosystem. Once infected, the fungus blocks the tree's water-conducting vessels, leading to wilting, yellowing leaves, and eventual death.

One of the most distinctive symptoms of Dutch Elm Disease is the wilting of leaves on individual branches, which progresses from the top of the tree downwards. As the disease progresses, the leaves turn yellow, then brown, and eventually fall off. The tree's bark may also display discoloration and exhibit signs of beetle activity, such as small entry holes or tunnels.

Preventing the spread of Dutch Elm Disease is crucial to preserve elm tree populations. Students can learn about various preventive measures, including sanitation practices and prompt removal of infected trees. Sanitation involves the removal and destruction of infected wood to eliminate the fungal spores and beetles that can spread the disease. Additionally, students can explore the importance of pruning and maintaining tree health to reduce vulnerability to infection.

Understanding the biology of the fungus and the beetle vectors is also essential in tackling Dutch Elm Disease. Students can dive into the life cycle and behavior of the Ophiostoma ulmi fungus and the various bark beetle species responsible for its transmission. This knowledge can help identify potential strategies to disrupt the disease's spread, such as targeted insecticide treatments or the use of resistant elm tree varieties.

Overall, learning about Dutch Elm Disease is vital for students interested in botany and plant pathology. By understanding the causes, symptoms, and prevention methods, students can contribute to the preservation of elm trees and the overall health of our ecosystems.

Citrus Canker

Citrus canker is a highly contagious and destructive plant disease that affects citrus trees worldwide. This subchapter will delve into the fascinating world of citrus canker, providing students with a comprehensive understanding of this plant pathology phenomenon.

1. Introduction to Citrus Canker: Citrus canker is caused by a bacterial pathogen called Xanthomonas citri subsp. citri. It primarily affects citrus trees, including oranges, lemons, limes, and grapefruits. This disease is characterized by raised corky lesions on the leaves, stems, and fruits of infected trees.

2. Life Cycle and Transmission: Understanding the life cycle and transmission of citrus canker is crucial to combat its spread. The bacteria enter the plant through natural openings or wounds, where they multiply and cause infections. Rain, wind, and human activities can also aid in the dispersal of the bacteria to healthy trees.

3. Symptoms and Diagnosis: Identifying the symptoms of citrus canker is essential for early detection and management. Students will learn to recognize the distinctive raised, corky lesions that appear on infected plants. Proper diagnosis involves laboratory tests, including microscopic examination and molecular techniques.

4. Impact on Citrus Industry: The citrus industry heavily relies on healthy trees for profitable yields. Citrus canker can devastate orchards, leading to economic losses and reduced fruit quality. Students will gain insights into the impact of this

disease on the citrus industry, and the importance of implementing control measures.

5.   Management   and   Prevention: Effective management strategies can help control and prevent the spread of citrus canker. Students will explore various techniques, including the removal and destruction of infected plant parts, chemical treatments, and the use of resistant cultivars. They will also learn about quarantine measures and strict regulations to prevent the disease's introduction in new areas.

6.   Global   Efforts   and   Research: Discover the worldwide efforts and ongoing research to combat citrus canker. Students will explore case studies highlighting successful control programs and the collaborative work of scientists, farmers, and government agencies in managing this disease.

Conclusion:
Citrus canker is a formidable enemy of the citrus industry, but armed with knowledge and effective management strategies, we can protect our beloved citrus trees. By understanding the life cycle, symptoms, and management techniques, students can become disease detectives, unraveling the secrets of plant pathology and contributing to the future of botany and agriculture.

Citrus canker is a highly contagious, bacterial disease that affects citrus plants, causing unsightly lesions on leaves, stems, and fruit. It is one of the most devastating diseases in the world of botany, posing a significant threat to the citrus industry worldwide.

The bacteria responsible for citrus canker is called Xanthomonas citri subsp. citri. It enters the plant through wounds or natural openings, such as stomata, and multiplies rapidly in the plant tissue, leading to the formation of raised corky lesions. These lesions can vary in size and shape, ranging from small, circular spots to larger, irregular-shaped areas.

One of the most concerning aspects of citrus canker is its ability to spread rapidly. The bacteria can be easily disseminated through wind-driven rain, insects, or even human activities, such as pruning or harvesting citrus fruits. Once a plant becomes infected, the bacteria can survive on the surface of the lesions for an extended period, making it difficult to control the disease.

Citrus canker affects the overall health of the citrus plant, weakening it and reducing its ability to produce healthy fruit. Infected fruit may drop prematurely, reducing both quality and yield. Additionally, the lesions on the fruit make it unattractive and unsuitable for commercial sale.

To control and manage citrus canker, various strategies are employed. These include cultural practices such as pruning infected plant material, disinfecting tools, and implementing strict sanitation measures. Chemical treatments are also used to reduce the spread of the disease, although they are not always the most sustainable option.

Awareness and education play a crucial role in preventing the spread of citrus canker. Students studying botany can contribute to the fight against this disease by learning to recognize the symptoms and understanding the importance of early detection. By being vigilant and reporting any suspected cases, they can help protect their own citrus plants and support efforts to prevent the disease from spreading further.

In conclusion, citrus canker is a significant threat to the citrus industry, causing devastating effects on plant health and fruit production. Understanding the biology of the disease, its symptoms, and management strategies is essential for students interested in botany. By learning about citrus canker, students can actively contribute to the prevention and control of this destructive plant pathology, ensuring the future of the citrus industry remains bright.

Success Stories in Disease Management

In the world of botany, disease management plays a crucial role in ensuring the health and survival of plants. Over the years, scientists and researchers have made significant advancements in the field of plant pathology, leading to numerous success stories in disease management. These success stories have not only helped in preventing and controlling plant diseases but also in safeguarding our food supply, preserving biodiversity, and promoting sustainable agriculture practices. Let's explore some of these remarkable success stories.

One of the most notable success stories in disease management is the control of the devastating disease called late blight in potatoes. Late blight, caused by the fungus Phytophthora infestans, was responsible for the infamous Irish potato famine in the 1840s. However, through extensive research and breeding programs, scientists have developed resistant potato varieties that can withstand this fungus. This breakthrough has not only saved countless potato crops but also minimized the need for chemical fungicides, promoting environmentally friendly farming practices.

Another success story revolves around the management of the citrus greening disease, also known as huanglongbing (HLB). HLB, caused by a bacterium called Candidatus Liberibacter asiaticus, has wreaked havoc on citrus orchards across the globe. However, scientists have developed early detection methods and implemented strict quarantine measures to prevent the spread of the disease. Additionally, researchers are exploring genetic engineering techniques to develop HLB-resistant citrus varieties, offering hope for the future of the citrus industry.

Furthermore, the successful management of the banana wilt disease in East Africa serves as an inspiring example. This disease, caused by the fungus Fusarium oxysporum f. sp. cubense, devastated banana plantations and threatened the staple food source for millions of people. Through the collaboration of scientists, farmers, and government agencies, a holistic approach was implemented, including the use of resistant banana varieties, cultural practices, and biocontrol agents. This integrated disease management strategy has significantly reduced the impact of banana wilt, ensuring food security and livelihoods for the affected communities.

These success stories highlight the importance of disease management in botany and the remarkable achievements made by scientists and researchers. As students of botany, it is crucial to understand the significance of these breakthroughs and their implications for sustainable agriculture and food security. By studying these success stories, we can gain valuable insights into the world of plant pathology and contribute to the ongoing efforts in disease management, ultimately ensuring a healthier and more resilient plant kingdom.

In the world of botany, disease management plays a crucial role in ensuring the health and productivity of plants. Over the years, scientists and researchers have made significant advancements in the field of plant pathology, leading to numerous success stories in disease management. These stories serve as a testament to the power of knowledge and innovation in overcoming challenges and protecting our plants.

One remarkable success story in disease management is the control of the devastating plant disease known as "late blight." Late blight is caused by a pathogen called Phytophthora infestans and is responsible for the infamous Irish potato famine in the mid-19th century. However, through extensive research and breeding efforts, scientists have developed resistant potato varieties that can withstand the onslaught of this destructive disease. This breakthrough has not only saved countless crops but also ensured food security for many regions around the world.

Another inspiring success story revolves around the management of the citrus greening disease, also known as Huanglongbing (HLB). HLB is a bacterial disease that affects citrus trees, causing a decline in fruit quality and yield. Scientists have been working tirelessly to combat this disease by developing innovative detection methods, implementing strict quarantine measures, and promoting the use of disease-resistant rootstocks. These efforts have proved successful in preventing the spread of HLB and protecting citrus industries worldwide.

Furthermore, biotechnological advancements have revolutionized disease management strategies. Genetic engineering techniques have enabled scientists to develop genetically modified (GM) crops with enhanced disease resistance. For instance, GM cotton varieties have been engineered to produce a toxin that kills specific insect pests, reducing the reliance on chemical pesticides and mitigating the spread of diseases transmitted by these pests.

Success stories in disease management highlight the importance of continuous research, collaboration, and innovative solutions in the field of plant pathology. They also serve as an inspiration to students interested in botany, providing them with real-life examples of how their knowledge and passion can make a difference in the world.

As students of botany, it is essential to stay updated with these success stories and learn from the strategies employed in disease management. By understanding the challenges faced and the innovative solutions developed, we can contribute to the future of agriculture and plant health.

In conclusion, success stories in disease management demonstrate the remarkable progress made in protecting plants from harmful pathogens. From developing disease-resistant varieties to implementing stringent quarantine measures and utilizing biotechnology, scientists have made significant strides in safeguarding our crops and ensuring food security. As students of botany, let us be inspired by these success stories and strive to contribute to the field of plant pathology by unraveling the secrets of disease management.

The Elimination of Rinderpest

Rinderpest, a highly contagious viral disease that affects cattle and other cloven-hoofed animals, has plagued the world for centuries. However, thanks to the efforts of dedicated scientists and veterinarians, this devastating disease has been successfully eradicated. In this subchapter, we will delve into the fascinating story of how rinderpest was eliminated, showcasing the significance of plant pathology in safeguarding the health of our planet's ecosystems.

Rinderpest, also known as cattle plague, caused immense suffering and economic losses throughout history. It spread rapidly, wiping out entire herds and leading to famine and economic collapse in many regions. However, through a combination of scientific research, international collaboration, and vaccination campaigns, rinderpest has become the first animal disease to be eradicated globally.

Plant pathology played a crucial role in the elimination of rinderpest. Scientists studying the disease recognized the importance of understanding its transmission and epidemiology. By investigating the virus's lifecycle, they were able to develop effective vaccines to protect animals from infection. These vaccines were then distributed worldwide, leading to widespread vaccination campaigns that ultimately halted the spread of the disease.

Students interested in botany will find that plant pathology intersects with the elimination of rinderpest in surprising ways. The disease, although primarily affecting animals, also had indirect effects on plants. During outbreaks, many farmers had to abandon their fields due to the loss of their livestock. This abandonment of agricultural land led to the invasion of weeds and the spread of plant diseases, further exacerbating the crisis. By eradicating rinderpest, plant pathology not only protected animals but also helped restore balance to ecosystems and promote sustainable agriculture.

The successful elimination of rinderpest serves as a testament to the power of scientific research, international collaboration, and proactive measures. It highlights the importance of early detection, prompt response, and vaccination programs in preventing the spread of infectious diseases. Students interested in botany can draw inspiration from this remarkable achievement and recognize the vital role that plant pathology plays in safeguarding the health of our planet.

In conclusion, the elimination of rinderpest stands as a milestone in the history of disease eradication. It showcases the profound impact of plant pathology in protecting both animals and plants. By studying the eradication of rinderpest, students can gain valuable insights into the complex interconnections between different branches of science and the role they play in addressing global challenges.

Rinderpest, also known as cattle plague, was a devastating viral disease that affected animals, particularly cattle and other cloven-hoofed animals. For centuries, it wreaked havoc on livestock populations, causing significant economic losses and threatening food security in many parts of the world. However, thanks to the efforts of scientists and veterinarians, rinderpest has been successfully eradicated, providing a remarkable example of the power of science in combating plant and animal diseases.

The journey towards the elimination of rinderpest began in the late 19th century when researchers started to understand the nature of the disease and its transmission. They discovered that rinderpest was caused by a virus that spread through direct contact, contaminated water, and even through the air. This knowledge paved the way for the development of vaccines and diagnostic tools that were crucial in controlling the disease.

One of the most significant breakthroughs in the fight against rinderpest was the development of a highly effective vaccine. This vaccine, made from weakened or inactivated forms of the virus, stimulated the immune system of animals, making them resistant to the disease. Mass vaccination campaigns were conducted in affected regions, leading to a significant reduction in rinderpest cases.

Another key aspect of the eradication efforts was the establishment of strict control measures. Infected animals were promptly isolated, and movement restrictions were put in place to prevent the spread of the virus. This required close collaboration between veterinarians, farmers, and government agencies to implement effective control strategies.

International cooperation played a crucial role in the elimination of rinderpest. Organizations such as the Food and Agriculture Organization of the United Nations (FAO) and the World Organization for Animal Health (OIE) worked together to coordinate global efforts, share knowledge and resources, and provide support to affected countries. This collective approach helped in monitoring the disease, coordinating vaccination campaigns, and ensuring that the virus did not re-emerge.

In 2011, after years of relentless efforts, the world celebrated the eradication of rinderpest. It was the first animal disease to be eradicated globally, and a significant milestone in the history of veterinary medicine. The elimination of rinderpest not only saved countless animal lives but also protected the livelihoods of farmers and ensured food security in many regions.

The successful elimination of rinderpest serves as a shining example of the power of science, international collaboration, and proactive measures in disease control. It highlights the importance of ongoing research, surveillance, and vaccination programs to prevent the resurgence of such devastating diseases.

As students interested in botany, it is crucial to understand the impact of plant and animal diseases on our ecosystems and food systems. The eradication of rinderpest provides an inspiring example of how scientific knowledge and cooperation can lead to the successful control and elimination of diseases, protecting both plants and animals. It is a testament to the dedication and perseverance of scientists and veterinarians who work tirelessly to ensure the health and well-being of our planet's biodiversity.

Controlling Wheat Rust

Wheat rust, a common fungal disease, has been a persistent threat to global food security for centuries. This subchapter will delve into the various methods employed by plant pathologists and farmers to combat this devastating plant disease.

Before we dive into the control measures, it is important to understand the nature of wheat rust. Wheat rust is caused by three species of fungi: Puccinia graminis, Puccinia triticina, and Puccinia striiformis. These fungi attack wheat plants, leading to reduced yield, poor grain quality, and even complete crop failure. The spores of these fungi are easily dispersed by wind, making it a significant challenge to control the disease.

One of the primary means of controlling wheat rust is through the use of resistant wheat varieties. Plant breeders have developed wheat cultivars that possess genetic resistance to specific rust species. By selectively breeding these resistant varieties, farmers can reduce the risk and impact of wheat rust outbreaks. This method not only helps in preventing the disease but also reduces the reliance on chemical interventions.

Chemical control measures are another strategy employed to manage wheat rust. Fungicides are used to protect wheat plants by preventing the growth and spread of the fungi. It is crucial to apply fungicides during the early stages of infection or as a preventive measure to maximize their efficacy. However, the use of chemical control should be judicious to minimize environmental impact and avoid the development of fungicide-resistant strains of the rust fungi.

Cultural practices also play a significant role in controlling wheat rust. Crop rotation, for instance, involves alternating the cultivation of wheat with non-host crops to disrupt the life cycle of the pathogen. This practice reduces the buildup of rust spores in the soil, decreasing the risk of infection in subsequent wheat crops.

Additionally, timely removal of infected plant debris and weeds can help prevent the spread of rust spores. These measures reduce the availability of alternate hosts and inhibit the survival and multiplication of the rust fungi.

Lastly, continuous monitoring and surveillance of wheat fields are crucial for early detection and prompt management of rust outbreaks. Plant pathologists and farmers regularly inspect crops for signs of infection, such as yellow-orange pustules on the leaves. Early detection allows for timely intervention, reducing the potential damage caused by the disease.

In conclusion, controlling wheat rust requires a comprehensive approach that encompasses the use of resistant wheat varieties, chemical control, cultural practices, and vigilant monitoring. By combining these strategies, plant pathologists and farmers can effectively manage this destructive disease, ensuring the health and productivity of wheat crops worldwide.

Wheat rust is a common fungal disease that affects wheat plants, causing significant losses in crop yield and quality. As budding botanists and plant enthusiasts, it is essential for students to understand the importance of controlling this destructive plant pathogen. In this subchapter, we will explore different strategies and techniques used in the field of plant pathology to combat wheat rust and protect our precious wheat crops.

1. Crop rotation: Rotating crops is an effective method to break the disease cycle of wheat rust. By alternating wheat with non-host plants, the pathogen's survival and reproduction are disrupted, reducing its impact on future wheat crops. This practice also helps to maintain soil fertility and minimize other pests and diseases.

2. Resistant varieties: Breeding resistant wheat varieties is a long-term and sustainable approach to controlling wheat rust. Scientists identify and breed wheat strains that possess natural resistance to specific rust pathogens. By growing resistant varieties, farmers can minimize the need for chemical interventions and reduce the risk of disease outbreaks.

3. Fungicides: When the disease pressure is high, fungicides can be used to control wheat rust. However, it is crucial to follow proper guidelines and safety protocols while using these chemical treatments. Integrated pest management practices encourage the judicious use of fungicides as a last resort, minimizing their impact on the environment.

4. Early detection and monitoring: Regular field inspections and monitoring are essential to detect wheat rust early. Students can learn to identify the characteristic symptoms of wheat rust, such as orange or reddish pustules on leaves, stems, and spikes. By reporting any signs of infection to the appropriate authorities, they can aid in timely interventions and prevent the disease from spreading.

5. Public awareness and education: Students can play a vital role in raising awareness about wheat rust and its control measures. By participating in community programs, workshops, and school initiatives, they can educate others about the importance of disease management practices and the impact of wheat rust on food security.

Understanding and controlling wheat rust is crucial for the future of agriculture and global food production. As students passionate about botany, learning about these strategies will equip you with the knowledge and skills to contribute to the field of plant pathology, ensuring the security of our food supply and the health of our crops. So let's dive into the fascinating world of wheat rust control and become disease detectives in the realm of botany!

Chapter 8: Future Directions in Plant Pathology

Emerging Challenges in Plant Disease Management

In the fascinating world of botany, the study of plants goes beyond their beauty and ecological importance. It delves into the intricate relationship between plants and the diseases that can threaten their survival. As students of botany, it is essential to understand the emerging challenges in plant disease management and the efforts made by disease detectives to unravel their secrets.

One of the major challenges in plant disease management is the constant evolution of plant pathogens. Just as humans face new strains of viruses, plants also encounter novel pathogens that have adapted to their environment. These pathogens can rapidly spread and cause devastating epidemics, posing a threat to crop production and ecosystem stability. Disease detectives, also known as plant pathologists, work tirelessly to identify and understand these emerging pathogens to develop effective management strategies.

Climate change is another critical challenge in plant disease management. Rising temperatures, altered precipitation patterns, and increased frequency of extreme weather events create favorable conditions for the proliferation of plant diseases. As botany students, it is crucial to recognize the role of climate change in altering disease dynamics and the urgency to find sustainable solutions.

Global trade and travel are also contributing to the emergence and spread of plant diseases. With the increase in international transportation, pathogens can hitch a ride on plants, seeds, or even soil, crossing borders and continents. This poses a significant challenge for disease detectives, as they must monitor and control the movement of such pathogens to prevent outbreaks in new regions.

The overuse of pesticides and the emergence of pesticide-resistant pathogens create yet another challenge in plant disease management. Prolonged and indiscriminate use of chemicals can lead to the development of resistant strains, rendering pesticides ineffective. Disease detectives are now focusing on integrated pest management strategies that combine cultural, biological, and chemical control methods, reducing reliance on pesticides and promoting sustainable practices.

Furthermore, the rapid expansion of urbanization and loss of natural habitats are impacting plant health. Urban environments, with their limited biodiversity and high levels of pollution, can stress plants, making them more susceptible to diseases. Disease detectives are exploring innovative solutions such as green roofs, vertical gardens, and urban farming to mitigate these challenges and enhance plant health in cities.

In conclusion, the field of plant pathology presents exciting challenges for students of botany. As emerging pathogens, climate change, global trade, pesticide resistance, and urbanization continue to pose threats to plant health, disease detectives play a crucial role in unraveling these secrets. By understanding these challenges and embracing sustainable practices, future botanists can become effective disease detectives, safeguarding the health and well-being of our precious plant species.

As students interested in botany, it is crucial to understand the emerging challenges in plant disease management. Plant pathology, the study of plant diseases, plays a vital role in maintaining global food security and the health of our ecosystem. However, with the ever-changing environment and globalization, new challenges are constantly arising.

One of the major emerging challenges in plant disease management is the spread of invasive species. Invasive pests and pathogens can easily be transported across continents through international trade and travel. As a result, previously isolated plant populations are now vulnerable to diseases they have never encountered before. This poses a significant threat to agricultural systems and natural ecosystems.

Climate change is another pressing challenge. Rising temperatures, altered precipitation patterns, and extreme weather events create favorable conditions for the spread and development of plant diseases. For instance, warmer winters enable pests and pathogens to survive in regions previously too cold for them, leading to the expansion of their range. Additionally, changes in rainfall patterns can affect the timing and intensity of disease outbreaks, making it harder to predict and manage them effectively.

Another challenge is the emergence of new strains of plant pathogens. Pathogens have the ability to evolve and adapt to their environment, making them more difficult to control. Genetic variation in pathogens can lead to the development of new strains that are more aggressive, resistant to treatments, or capable of infecting previously resistant plant varieties. This necessitates constant monitoring and research to keep up with the evolving nature of plant diseases.

Furthermore, the increasing use of pesticides and fungicides has unintended consequences. Prolonged and intensive use of these chemicals can lead to the development of pesticide-resistant pathogens and harmful effects on beneficial organisms, such as pollinators and soil microorganisms. As future botanists, it is essential to explore alternative methods of disease management, such as integrated pest management and biological control, to minimize the negative impacts of chemical control measures.

In conclusion, the field of plant pathology is facing numerous emerging challenges that require innovative approaches to disease management. The spread of invasive species, climate change, the emergence of new strains, and the unintended consequences of chemical control measures all pose significant threats to plant health. As students interested in botany, it is our responsibility to stay informed about these challenges and actively contribute to finding sustainable solutions. By understanding and addressing these emerging challenges, we can ensure the health and vitality of plants, agriculture, and ecosystems for future generations.

Advances in Technology and Research

In the ever-evolving field of botany, technological advancements have revolutionized the way researchers study and understand plant pathology. These breakthroughs have paved the way for exciting discoveries and have opened up new avenues for students interested in exploring the secrets of plant diseases. This subchapter will delve into some of the most impactful advances in technology and research, highlighting their significance in the field of botany.

One of the key advancements is the use of DNA sequencing techniques. Scientists can now decode the entire genetic makeup of plants, allowing them to identify specific genes responsible for disease resistance or susceptibility. This has led to the development of genetically modified crops that can withstand diseases, reducing the need for harmful pesticides and increasing food production. Students interested in botany can now explore the world of genetic engineering and contribute to the development of disease-resistant crops.

Another significant advancement is the use of remote sensing technologies. Satellites equipped with advanced sensors can collect data on plant health and growth from space. By analyzing this data, scientists can detect early signs of diseases and monitor their spread. This technology has proven invaluable in large-scale crop management, enabling timely interventions to prevent widespread damage. Students can now learn how to interpret satellite images and contribute to the monitoring of plant diseases on a global scale.

Furthermore, advancements in microscopy have allowed scientists to observe plant pathogens at a microscopic level. High-resolution imaging techniques provide detailed insights into the structure and behavior of these pathogens, aiding in the development of targeted treatments. Students can now explore the fascinating world of microscopic organisms and contribute to the development of innovative strategies to combat plant diseases.

Lastly, the field of data analytics has revolutionized the way researchers analyze and interpret large datasets. By using sophisticated algorithms, scientists can identify patterns and correlations in complex datasets, leading to better disease prediction and management strategies. Students with a knack for data analysis can now apply their skills to unravel the secrets of plant pathology.

In conclusion, advances in technology and research have greatly enhanced our understanding of plant pathology. Students interested in botany now have the opportunity to explore exciting fields such as genetic engineering, remote sensing, microscopy, and data analytics. By embracing these advancements, the next generation of disease detectives can unravel the secrets of plant pathology and contribute to the sustainable and healthy future of our planet.

In the ever-evolving field of plant pathology, breakthroughs in technology and research have revolutionized the way we study and combat plant diseases. These advances have not only enhanced our understanding of plant pathology but also provided promising solutions to safeguard our precious botanical resources. In this subchapter, we will explore some of the remarkable advancements that are driving the field forward.

One of the most significant advancements in plant pathology is the utilization of cutting-edge technologies. For instance, DNA sequencing techniques have allowed researchers to identify and characterize plant pathogens with unprecedented accuracy. By studying the genetic makeup of pathogens, scientists can better understand their behavior, transmission, and potential impact on plant health. This knowledge is instrumental in developing targeted strategies to prevent and control diseases.

Furthermore, advanced imaging technologies have transformed the way we visualize and study plant diseases. Microscopes equipped with high-resolution cameras enable researchers to capture detailed images of infected plant tissues, aiding in the identification of specific pathogens and the assessment of disease progression. Additionally, remote sensing techniques, such as satellite imagery and drones, provide a holistic view of disease outbreaks across vast agricultural landscapes, allowing for timely interventions and mitigation measures.

Another exciting area of advancement in plant pathology research is genetic engineering. Scientists are now able to manipulate the genetic makeup of plants to enhance their resistance to diseases. By introducing genes that produce antimicrobial compounds or activate defense mechanisms, researchers can develop disease-resistant crop varieties that withstand even the most virulent pathogens. This breakthrough in genetic engineering holds immense promise for sustainable agriculture and food security.

Moreover, the integration of big data analytics and artificial intelligence has revolutionized disease monitoring and prediction. Through the analysis of vast amounts of data, including climatic conditions, plant health records, and disease prevalence, researchers can develop models and algorithms that forecast disease outbreaks. This early warning system allows farmers and policymakers to take proactive measures to prevent or mitigate the spread of diseases, minimizing economic losses and environmental impact.

As students of botany, these advancements in technology and research offer exciting opportunities to explore the fascinating world of plant pathology. By embracing these tools and knowledge, we can contribute to the development of innovative solutions and strategies to protect our plants and ecosystems. The future of botany and plant pathology is undoubtedly intertwined with the advancements we have discussed, and by staying at the forefront of these developments, we can unravel the secrets of plant diseases and ensure a sustainable future for our botanical world.

Careers in Plant Pathology

If you are passionate about plants and have a keen interest in understanding and combating plant diseases, a career in plant pathology might be just what you're looking for. Plant pathology is a branch of botany that focuses on the study of plant diseases, their causes, and ways to prevent or control them. In this subchapter, we will explore the exciting and diverse careers available in the field of plant pathology.

One of the most common career paths for plant pathologists is that of a plant disease diagnostician. These professionals work in laboratories, botanical gardens, or agricultural research centers, where they analyze plant samples to identify diseases and develop appropriate treatment plans. As a diagnostician, you will get to solve puzzles by observing symptoms, conducting tests, and using advanced technologies to determine the cause of plant diseases.

Another fascinating career option is that of a plant disease researcher. These scientists work in universities, government agencies, or private research firms, where they conduct experiments and studies to gain a deeper understanding of plant diseases. By studying the biology, genetics, and ecology of plant pathogens, researchers contribute to the development of new strategies for disease management and crop improvement.

If you have a passion for teaching and sharing knowledge, a career as a plant pathology professor might be your calling. Professors in this field work in universities, where they educate and train the next generation of plant pathologists. They also conduct research and contribute to scientific advancements in the field.

For those interested in the interface between plant pathology and technology, a career as a bioinformatics specialist may be a perfect fit. These professionals develop computer algorithms and tools to analyze and interpret large datasets generated from plant disease research. Bioinformatics experts play a crucial role in understanding the complex interactions between plants, pathogens, and the environment.

Lastly, if you enjoy working directly with farmers and growers, a career as an agricultural extension specialist could be a great choice. Extension specialists provide advice and guidance to farmers on disease prevention and management strategies. They also conduct workshops, deliver presentations, and publish informative materials to educate the agricultural community about the latest developments in plant pathology.

In conclusion, plant pathology offers a range of exciting and rewarding career opportunities for students interested in the field of botany. Whether you prefer laboratory work, research, teaching, technology, or hands-on interactions with farmers, there is a career path in plant pathology that suits your interests and skills. So, if you have a passion for plants and a desire to unravel the secrets of plant diseases, consider pursuing a career in plant pathology and become a disease detective yourself!

If you have a passion for botany and a curiosity for uncovering the secrets of plant diseases, a career in plant pathology might be the perfect fit for you. Plant pathology is a fascinating field of study that focuses on understanding and managing plant diseases, which can have a significant impact on agriculture, the environment, and human health.

As a plant pathologist, you will be at the forefront of investigating and identifying the causes of plant diseases. Your work will involve studying the interactions between plants, pathogens, and the environment to develop strategies for disease prevention, control, and management. You will also play a crucial role in preserving crop yield and quality, ensuring food security, and protecting natural ecosystems.

There are various exciting career paths within the field of plant pathology. One option is to become a research scientist, where you can work in academic or government institutions, conducting cutting-edge research to advance our understanding of plant diseases. By studying the molecular biology, genetics, and ecology of plant pathogens, you will contribute to the development of innovative solutions to combat these diseases.

Another career option is to work as a diagnostician or plant disease detective. In this role, you will investigate and diagnose plant diseases in the field or laboratory. By identifying the specific pathogens causing the diseases, you will help farmers and growers implement effective control measures, ultimately improving crop yields and reducing economic losses.

Plant pathology also offers opportunities in the field of plant breeding and genetics. As a plant pathologist working in this area, you will develop disease-resistant varieties of crops through traditional breeding techniques or genetic engineering. By creating plants that are resilient to diseases, you will contribute to sustainable agriculture and food production.

Furthermore, plant pathologists can also find rewarding careers in plant quarantine and biosecurity. In this role, you will be responsible for preventing the introduction and spread of plant diseases across borders. By implementing strict regulations and protocols, you will safeguard agricultural industries and protect native plant species from invasive pathogens.

In conclusion, a career in plant pathology offers a world of opportunities for students with a passion for botany. Whether you choose to become a research scientist, diagnostician, plant breeder, or work in plant quarantine, your work will be crucial in understanding, managing, and ultimately preventing the devastating effects of plant diseases. By pursuing a career in plant pathology, you will contribute to the sustainable future of agriculture and make a positive impact on our environment and society.

Chapter 9: Conclusion and Key Takeaways

Recap of Key Concepts

In our journey to unravel the secrets of plant pathology, we have covered several key concepts that are fundamental to understanding the world of botany and disease detection. This recap will serve as a valuable resource for students to review and reinforce their knowledge.

One of the primary concepts we explored is the importance of plant health. We learned that plants, just like humans, can fall sick and require proper care and attention. Understanding the signs and symptoms of plant diseases is crucial for early detection and effective treatment. By closely observing changes in leaf color, wilting, or unusual growth patterns, we can identify potential issues and take immediate action.

Another vital concept is the role of pathogens in plant diseases. We delved into the world of bacteria, fungi, viruses, and other microorganisms that can harm plants. We learned how these pathogens invade plant tissues, multiply, and disrupt the normal functioning of plants. Students also gained an understanding of how pathogens spread through various means, such as wind, water, insects, or contaminated soil.

To combat plant diseases, we explored the concept of integrated pest management (IPM). This holistic approach emphasizes a combination of preventive measures, cultural practices, biological controls, and judicious use of chemical treatments. By implementing IPM strategies, students can learn how to maintain healthy plants while minimizing the environmental impact.

In our exploration of plant pathology, we also discussed the importance of plant resistance and breeding for disease resistance. Students learned that some plant varieties possess natural resistance against specific pathogens, while others can be bred to develop resistance. Understanding the principles of plant breeding allows students to contribute to the development of disease-resistant crops, ensuring food security and sustainable agriculture.

Lastly, we reviewed the techniques used by disease detectives, the plant pathologists, in diagnosing and studying plant diseases. From conducting laboratory tests to utilizing advanced tools like DNA sequencing, microscopy, and imaging, students were introduced to the fascinating world of scientific research and investigation.

By revisiting these key concepts, students can solidify their understanding of plant pathology and its significance in the field of botany. Armed with this knowledge, they will be better equipped to identify, prevent, and manage plant diseases, contributing to a healthier and more sustainable future for our plant kingdom.

As we reach the end of this chapter, it's important to recap the key concepts we have covered so far. Understanding these concepts will not only help you grasp the fundamental principles of plant pathology but also equip you with the knowledge to become a skilled disease detective in the field of botany.

Firstly, we explored the basics of plant pathology, which is the study of plant diseases. We learned about the different types of pathogens that can attack plants, such as bacteria, fungi, viruses, and nematodes. Understanding the nature of these pathogens is crucial in identifying and managing plant diseases effectively.

Next, we delved into the symptoms and signs exhibited by plants when they are infected by pathogens. We discussed the various symptoms, including wilting, discoloration, necrosis, and stunting, and how these signs can help in diagnosing the disease. We also emphasized the importance of early detection to prevent further spread and damage to plants.

We then moved on to exploring the ways in which plant diseases can spread. Understanding the modes of transmission is crucial in developing effective disease management strategies. We discussed the role of vectors, such as insects and wind, as well as the significance of contaminated soil, water, and infected seeds in spreading diseases.

Furthermore, we delved into the concept of plant immunity and resistance. We learned about the defense mechanisms that plants have developed to protect themselves from pathogens. We discussed the role of physical barriers, chemical responses, and genetic resistance in preventing or minimizing the impact of diseases.

Lastly, we touched upon the importance of integrated pest management (IPM) in disease control. IPM involves a combination of various strategies, including cultural, biological, and chemical methods, to manage plant diseases effectively while minimizing environmental harm.

In conclusion, this chapter has provided you with a comprehensive overview of the key concepts in plant pathology. By understanding the types of pathogens, symptoms, modes of transmission, plant immunity, and disease management strategies, you are now equipped with the fundamental knowledge to become a successful disease detective in the field of botany. Keep exploring, asking questions, and applying the concepts you have learned to unravel the secrets of plant pathology.

Importance of Plant Pathology for Sustainable Agriculture

In the world of plant pathology, understanding the different diseases that can affect plants is crucial for maintaining healthy crops and gardens. This subchapter, titled "Index," is designed to help students navigate through the vast amount of information contained in this book, "Disease Detectives: Unraveling the Secrets of Plant Pathology for Students," with a focus on the niche of botany.

The index serves as a valuable tool for students to quickly locate specific topics within the book. It is organized alphabetically, making it easy to find information on particular diseases, pathogens, or plant species. In addition, the index includes cross-references, directing students to related topics or concepts that may be of interest.

For students studying botany, this index will prove particularly beneficial. It provides a comprehensive list of plant diseases, including fungal, bacterial, and viral pathogens that can harm various plant species. Whether it's learning about the symptoms of a specific disease or understanding the lifecycle of a pathogen, the index will guide students to the relevant sections in the book.

Furthermore, the index also includes terms and concepts related to botany and plant pathology. From terms like "photosynthesis" and "plant anatomy" to more specific topics such as "host resistance" and "phytopathogenic fungi," students will find a wealth of information to deepen their understanding of plant biology and disease detection.

To enhance the learning experience, the index is accompanied by page numbers, enabling students to quickly locate the desired content within the book. This feature facilitates efficient study sessions, making it easier for students to review specific topics or refer back to information they have previously read.

In conclusion, the "Index" subchapter of "Disease Detectives: Unraveling the Secrets of Plant Pathology for Students" provides a valuable tool for students studying botany and interested in plant pathology. By organizing the content alphabetically and providing cross-references, students can easily navigate through the book, locate specific topics, and expand their knowledge of plant diseases. Whether you are researching a particular pathogen or seeking a better understanding of plant biology, this index will be an indispensable resource on your journey to becoming a disease detective in the fascinating world of botany.

In Disease Detectives: Unraveling the Secrets of Plant Pathology for Students, the index serves as a valuable tool to help you navigate through the wealth of information contained within this book. As budding botany enthusiasts, it is essential to have a comprehensive reference at your fingertips, allowing you to quickly locate specific topics, terms, and concepts related to plant pathology.

The index is organized alphabetically, making it easy for you to find what you're looking for. Whether you want to understand the symptoms of a particular plant disease, learn about the various pathogens that affect plants, or explore the methods used by disease detectives to identify and control plant diseases, the index has you covered.

For instance, if you're interested in learning about fungal diseases, simply flip to the "F" section in the index, and you'll find a list of pages dedicated to fungal pathogens such as rusts, powdery mildews, and blights. Each entry in the index is accompanied by a brief description, giving you a glimpse into the topic covered on that page.

Additionally, the index includes cross-references, ensuring that you don't miss any related information. For example, if you're reading about aphids and want to know more about the specific plants they target, you can refer to the cross-reference that will lead you to the appropriate page.

The index also serves as a tool for reviewing and revisiting specific topics. If you're studying for an exam or working on a research project, you can use the index to quickly locate relevant pages and refresh your memory on key concepts.

Overall, the index in Disease Detectives: Unraveling the Secrets of Plant Pathology for Students is an indispensable resource for students of botany. It provides a roadmap to navigate the fascinating world of plant diseases, ensuring that you can easily access the information you need. Whether you're a beginner or an advanced student, this index will enable you to dive deep into the captivating field of plant pathology and become a skilled disease detective.